The Really Useful Teenage Food Guide

The Really Useful Teenage Food Guide

Healthy ways to eat well
and feel great
– without dieting

Janette Marshall

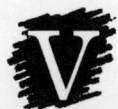

V

VERMILION

First published in 1996

1 3 5 7 9 10 8 6 4 2

Copyright © Janette Marshall 1996

Janette Marshall has asserted her right to be identified as the author of this work.

First published in the United Kingdom in 1996 by Vermilion
an imprint of Ebury Press
Random House · 20 Vauxhall Bridge Road · London SW1V 2SA

Random House Australia (Pty) Limited
20 Alfred Street · Milsons Point · Sydney · New South Wales 2061 · Australia

Random House New Zealand Limited
18 Poland Road · Glenfield · Auckland 10 · New Zealand

Random House South Africa (Pty) Limited
PO Box 2263 · Rosebank 2121 · South Africa

Random House UK Limited Reg. No. 954009

A CIP catalogue record for this book is available from the British Library.

ISBN: 0 09 181 468 5

Printed and bound in Great Britain by Mackays of Chatham plc.

Papers used by Vermilion are natural, recyclable
products made from wood grown in sustainable forest.

Contents

How to use this book

During the teens adolescents gradually take more and more decisions for themselves, yet it is often parents who face the day-to-day practicalities such as food preparation (shopping and cooking) – and do the worrying! This book addresses both teenagers and parents. Some chapters are addressed more directly to teenagers and some to parents. For example, there are quizzes for teenagers in chapter 8, and there is advice for parents on healthy eating for vegetarians in chapter 7 and how to spot potential problems such as eating disorders in chapter 6. While there is nothing to stop either party reading the entire book, it might be useful to know which chapters are specifically aimed at which readers.

Teenagers: chapter 8

Parents: chapters 1, 6, 7

Both: chapters 2, 3, 4, 5, 9

Teenagers this symbol indicates a special message for you.

Parents this symbol highlights practical ways to make changes for the better.

Introduction

'...it has never been easier to eat well in Britain, but too many of our children are either starving themselves to emulate stick-insect models, or turning into couch potatoes on a diet of chips and Coca-Cola...'
Daily Telegraph, October 1995.

Teenage diets are far from ideal. Many are not even adequate, and they are without doubt storing up trouble for the future.

In fact teenage eating habits are a potential time bomb, with explosive consequences for health as adults, and far-reaching effects on the health of future generations.

The typical eating pattern is one of replacing meals with snacks throughout the day, or supplementing poor quality meals with crisps, sweets, chocolate and fizzy drinks.

Most adolescents rely on a very limited number of foods. Virtually all are failing to meet current healthy eating recommendations, eating too much fatty and sugary food at the expense of more nutritious vegetables, fruit and energy-giving starchy high-fibre foods.

A worryingly large number go to school or college without having eaten breakfast. Lunch is a snack on the move. And while most eat a cooked meal after school, college or work, snacks still continue throughout the evening – with or without alcohol.

The diet of teenage girls, an increasing number of whom are smokers, is a cause for concern, and as the quotation above shows, the teenage habit of slimming is a cause of tension. On the one hand teenagers are being encouraged to change their eating habits to adopt a healthier diet. On the other hand parents worry when a teenage girl in particular starts to manipulate her food, or go on a slimming diet, lest she develop a slimming disorder such as anorexia nervosa. The aim of this book is to help teenagers and parents get the balance right (see chapter 6). Girls' daily diets often leave them tired, washed out and anaemic; those who are vegetarian are most at risk. If teenage girls carry on eating like this, there will be serious implications for their health as adults and for the health of the children they will have.

Given the poor state of many teenagers' diets it is hardly surprising that as a group they are not energetic enough to take exercise to become fit or to prevent future weight and health problems.

Why are teenagers eating so badly?

The majority of teenagers are, in fact, just following the example of adults throughout the developed world. They eat what adults eat and what adults provide for them to eat.

The poor diet of the British is now so serious a matter that diet and nutrition have been identified as a key target in reducing the high incidence of some of the western world's major public health problems such as heart disease, and cancer. Heart disease is still the main cause of death in Britain today, and stroke is a problem. While such disease is rare among young people, the eating habits of adolescence contribute to its onset later in life, and to high blood pressure, osteoporosis and obesity. What teenagers (and others) eat is also responsible for the fact that half of British adults are overweight or obese.

The aims of the changes to the British diet, to promote healthier eating, are to:

- reduce the proportion of British adults who are obese by at least 25% and 33% respectively by 2005 to no more than 6% of men and 8% of women
- reduce the contribution of fat to the diet from around 40% to no more than 35% of total food energy
- of that 35% fat, ensure that no more than 11% is from saturated fats

- reduce the contribution of sugar to the diet to no more than 11% of total energy
- reduce the proportion of men drinking more than 21 units of alcohol per week and women drinking more than 14 units per week by 30% to 18% of men and 7% of women

How do teenagers measure up?

The majority of teenagers are not eating anything like a well-balanced diet:

- about 75% of teenagers are eating more fat than they should
- the main sources of calories in a typical teenage diet are cakes, biscuits, meat products, puddings, chips, bread and milk (there's nothing wrong with the last two)
- intakes of B vitamins, calcium and, in particular, iron are far too low in teenage girls

This means that if teenagers do not radically change their diet, the futures of many may be cut short and they could end up adding to the heart disease and cancer mortality statistics well before their time.

Living for now

If long term health prospects are not of interest to you, and you are, quite rightly, more keen on having fun now than worrying about your long-term prospects, it's worth considering that eating a better diet now will give you more energy and vitality to live life to the full. A poor diet during the teen years means you will be undernourished (but possibly over-fed and overweight). You

- may not look as good as you could
- may feel too tired to enjoy yourself
- may end up with false teeth in your twenties
- may not reach your full growth potential
- may not reach your full academic potential
- may jeopardise your bone development

These are not exaggerations.

Nibbling away at our social foundations

There is a view that teenagers' eating habits are somehow subversive and contributing to a moral decline in society! In an era of unease about a perceived decline in moral standards and lack of social cohesion within and without the family, there is a popular idea that teenagers are undermining family life by taking solitary snacks, or 'grazing' throughout the day, rather than sitting down with the family each day for a 'proper' meal.

They are not the only ones. The members of most 'families' (or households) eat separately during the day (at home, school/college or work) and often eat in shifts when they are at home, to fit round leisure activities. If it is a two-parent household, mum and dad may be at work all or part of the day. Daytime meals may be snacks and packed or canteen lunches. After school, children may eat with a childminder, or with mum, or parents may eat together later in the evening after children have gone to bed. And the dining table may have become an arm chair in front of the tv.

In many cases, home-cooking has been replaced by convenience meals reheated in a microwave oven. And the skill of food preparation and cooking may no longer be taught in the home or the school. None of this is the fault of teenagers.

Blaming the 'stick insect' models

While some teenagers are possibly over-fed and undernourished, a minority may be underfed and under-nourished. These are the slimmers who attempt to become like their perceived ideal body image of a supermodel. Studies show that teenagers do over-estimate their body size after being shown magazines containing fashion pictures using waif-like models targetted at their age group. This inevitably makes them more likely to go on a slimming diet. However, for the majority of teenage girls dieting is a 'normal' part

of adolescence. While it is not to be encouraged, it does not always have unhealthy consequences, and it will not cause eating disorders such as anorexia nervosa which are something quite separate from 'normal'
teenage slimming activities (see chapter 6). Parents should not be unduly worried when teenage girls go on a diet, and an immediate heavy reaction against slimming may cause unnecessary confrontations. Instead parents could use the interest shown in food to initiate a change in the teenagers' (and if necessary, the whole family's) eating habits to adopt a healthier diet. Eating such a diet would obviate the need to 'slim', especially in the case of those teenage girlss who do not really need to lose weight.

An interest in slimming can start well before the teens and surveys show half of 11- and 12-year-old girls are concerned about their body shape and weight.

So what?

Why should this be of any concern? Because good diet and exercise are vitally important to teenagers and are an essential part of growing up. The enormous physical changes that happen during adolescence, and the equally important intellectual and emotional changes, mean teenage minds and bodies need to be properly fed and exercised.

If teenagers are to reach full physical and mental potential and optimum health they need to eat a well-balanced diet. This is crucial for healthy development, for functioning properly on a daily basis – and as an insurance policy for health later in life.

During the teens there occurs the major growth spurt that brings about rapid increases in height and weight, sexual maturation and many other changes in the body. These changes make large demands for energy and foods rich in vitamins and minerals which a poor diet cannot supply. Teenagers need to eat the right foods in the right proportions in order to have the energy to cope with all the changes, demands and stresses of adolescence.

Stone Age teenagers...

Today's teenagers are no different, in some respects, from their Stone Age ancestors! Which is not to say all teenagers are smelly and grungy with bedrooms that are as dirty and gloomy as caves, or that they are genetically programmed to be aggressive, uncouth and terminally unsophisticated – whatever parents may think. This is simply referring to inbuilt appetites.

In prehistoric times food was scarce and people tended to eat a lot when the chance arose. In evolutionary terms those of us with a hearty appetite survived. Healthy teenagers today have not changed much – parents who complain about the flocks of teenage gannets that raid their fridges, and then lie gorged and soporific around the home, will testify to this.

Like today's teenagers, Stone Age people had sharp appetites for fatty and sugary foods which were then scarce, and nutritionally inoffensive compared with a diet composed entirely of chocolate, burgers, sweet fizzy drinks and crisps. Today teenagers are surrounded by fatty and sugary snack foods – which profit-motivated 'adults' are keen to supply – so it's no wonder that some may over-eat them. Unfortunately, fatty and sugary foods are high in calories and low in the vitamins and minerals needed for health and vitality.

There's another Stone Age trait that also inhibits 'healthy eating' in the teens. It's called the Omnivore's Paradox, and is manifested from the toddler years to the teenage years. It seems designed to drive parents crazy.

I don't like it, mum...

What is the Omnivore's Paradox? Humans are naturally keen to try new foods but afraid of the consequences of eating something unknown. After all, trying a newly discovered berry or plant could have been fatal in the Stone Age. Today the reluctance to try new foods and the innate conservatism of toddlers and children can result in limited faddy diets which some have still not grown out of by the teenage years!

Of course it is not all due to genetics. Children and teenagers can and do learn to enjoy new foods. But often the trepidation with which parents offer new foods increases the problem. Who has not said, or heard said: 'You're not going to like this, but it's good for you, so eat it up'?

But can parents complain if they have used (knowingly or unknowingly) sweets, biscuits, cakes, crisps and fizzy drinks as rewards or to 'bribe' children, and made eating up their greens part of a punishment? With adults promulgating such attitudes, or taking the line of least resistance at meal times, or (even worse) expecting children to Eat as I Say, but Not as I Eat, it is no wonder that teenagers' diets leave a lot to be desired.

With a natural propensity to eat sugary and fatty foods, with newly found independence and money in their pockets, most teenagers will choose non-nutritious snacks, especially as British streets are peppered with fast food outlets, confectioners, tobacconists and convenience stores. It is all too easy for teenagers to eat 'junk' food everytime they feel hungry to the exclusion of healthier food like fruit, vegetables and bread.

Schools are not doing any better

Even in schools and colleges it may be impossible for teenagers to eat wisely. Most school meals provide far too many fatty foods, and since the abolition of nutritional standards and the imposition of the cash cafeteria system and compulsory tendering for the provision of school meals, the diets of teenagers have not improved. The high street alternatives to school meals are even worse, and tuck shops sell mainly confectionery and savoury snacks.

If the majority of children are eating 'junk' food, then peer pressure will ensure that the lowest common denominator in dietary terms prevails. While teenagers may rebel against parental and other authority figures, they often conform to peer pressure (starting at nursery school). And as food is a sign of friendship, what teenagers eat is determined by wherever the group decides is the right place to meet.

In general this will be in burger, chicken and pizza restaurants, plus pub 'restaurants' and fish and chip shops. Virtually all of these food outlets lack 'healthy options' on the menu. This would not normally be a problem, except that teenagers are the age group that most frequently 'eats out' and routinely uses the fast food chains in particular.

Although many households have made a general shift towards 'healthier eating' (changing to semi-skimmed milk, grilling instead of frying, cutting off visible fat, using fats low in saturates), teenagers are not necessarily 'safe' in their own homes. From nappies to puberty (or at least since they were toddlers) they are bombarded with advertising for junk food on children's tv.

Big business is out to get teenagers

The food industry spends a fortune developing, advertising and marketing food and drink products to appeal to young people. They talk about generating child appeal; they design brands to appeal to children and especially teenagers who have real spending power. They are out to build brand loyalty in children and exploit their eating habits for all they are worth – too often without a word or a passing nod to concerns for the nutritional status or health of the children.

Even pantomimes no longer retain their innocence, sponsored as they are by chocolate companies. And at major sporting events sponsored by soft drink and confectionery companies, entry may be refused to children carrying bottles of water or fruit juice or their own healthier food. Teenagers (and toddlers) are seen as fair game (or prey) by the multinationals.

Getting them hooked young is the aim, especially the aim of major (alcoholic) drinks' companies who have rightly received a bad press for introducing alcoholic lemonade, water and other soft drinks. In an age when we frown on the days when the wet nurse soaked a comforter cloth in gin, our morals seem rather confused. In the face of blatant and outrageous marketing of alcohol to children the government seems not to act in the interests of young people. Instead there is a reliance on ineffectual voluntary guidelines, while teenagers swig alcoholic cherryade on the streets.

Sitting targets

Teenagers have also been brought up to be less active! Many teenagers will have been placed in front of the tv (as toddlers), some would say to save parents and carers the effort of having to play with them or be active with them. Schools tell children to sit still and be quiet. From the earliest age, natural ebullience and love of movement are knocked out of children.

This might seem an exaggeration, and of course there would be chaos trying to teach physics to a class full of children charging around like a herd of cattle. But the point is that children's spontaneous delight in physical activity is stifled. School sports and physical education have the effect of putting many kids off physical activity. Parents take children to school and collect them by car – it is not considered safe for children to walk or cycle. With an emphasis on the academic and league tables in schools, teachers are forced to cut down on the physical activities. There are fewer team games at higher (aerobic) intensity. By the early teens nearly all girls and most boys have adopted the sedentary habits of a lifetime.

Erratic eating habits

Diet needs to be seen in perspective, in conjunction with all the other things going on during adolescence, which roughly corresponds to the teenage years. During the teen years there are complex physical, emotional, personality and psychological developments, bringing with them upheaval and change for the individual and the teenager's family.

Relationships change between teenagers and their parents, who will no longer tolerate childish behaviour. There is the need to identify the direction of career and further education. There is often conflict as teenagers demand more independence than parents think they are ready for.

Adolescence is a time of rebellion and experimentation. And one of the easiest ways of rebelling is to refuse to eat family foods, or make a statement of individuality by changing to, for example, a vegetarian diet. Vegetarianism is not in itself a problem, as long as it is done correctly (see chapter 7).

It's hardly surprising that at a time of emotional and intellectual turbulence, food intake may become erratic and food fads common. Lifestyle becomes less formal and structured as adolescents gain more independence and organise their own time. It is only natural that this results in a tendency to eat more snack meals or graze, neither of which need be hazardous if done properly (see 28 Day Healthy Eating Plan, chapter 4).

At the time of the teenage growth spurt, food is directly linked to changes in physical shape and size; worries about physical appearance and attractiveness are common. If these are handled insensitively or in an environment that does not allow expression of emotions and feelings with much-needed support, or if undue pressures are put on teenagers, there is the risk of individuals seeking 'solace' in food and becoming overweight or of developing an excessive interest in slimming. Girls especially are at risk of developing anorexia nervosa and possibly bulimia nervosa (see chapter 6).

The major food concerns of most teenagers are that what they eat should taste good and that it should not make them fat. Most consider that if they enjoy what they eat and are currently healthy then their diet must be harmless making it difficult to interest teenagers in the future effects of their present eating habits. Like so many adults, it is hard to get them to swallow that what they eat today may contribute to heart disease, bowel problems, cancer and other ills later in life.

Keep talking

Throughout all this upheaval and change, the most important thing is to maintain communication between parents and teenagers. It's not always easy, especially if adolescents are feeling alienated. The best thing for parents to do is stick to practical advice, without using any emotional influence. And don't despair – even minor changes can bring about big improvements (see teenager's food diaries in the next chapter).

The most valuable things a parent can do are:

- be a good role model, (what are your attitudes/actions on dieting for example?) and provide regular nourishing meals and snacks
- make sure teenagers eat breakfast (even if they take it with them)
- promote better snacking habits (chapter 5, The good snack guide) and provide alternatives to fizzy drinks
- encourage teenagers to eat daily fruit and vegetables (concentrating first on the ones they like)
- with girls, who may be vulnerable to excessive slimming, do not use the over-simplified healthy eating messages given to adults (eg that high fat foods and sugar are bad), because this can lead to girls avoiding important foods and rejecting or over-emphasising whole food groups
- however, take a relaxed attitude to 'normal' dieting and most important of all, don't go into battle with teenagers over food.

CHAPTER 1

Teenagers' food diaries

At the same time as having busy lives, a widening social scene and other demands that take precedence over joining in with family meals (where they exist), teenagers often have large appetites and eat voraciously. While some teenagers eat in an apparently indiscriminate way, for others what they eat is a matter of principle which leads to, for example, vegetarianism, or to a rejection of meat other than that produced to animal welfare standards, or to special diets prescribed by other ethical or environmental concerns.

Rejecting foods that are said to be 'good for you' by parents and other figures of authority is a normal part of adolescence. And even if teenagers are interested in healthy eating for the sake of their appearance or for sports training, other factors influence what they eat and drink. Food and drink has to have the right image, conform to peer group 'norms', be acceptable for sharing as snack foods and be affordable.

Tastes and food preferences can be as changeable and unpredictable as teenagers' moods. Indeed, not since the turmoil and tantrums of the toddler years has food been such an issue as it becomes for some teenagers. Or, so it seems to many parents.

This can be very irritating because teenagers need to eat a nutrient-dense diet. Nutrient-dense foods are those that provide more vitamins and minerals per mouthful than 'junk' foods which are mainly fat and sugar. Yet, as we will see, teenagers are frequently eating foods high in calories (fat and sugar) and low in vitamins and

---

Sugar – the facts

There are two types of sugar: 1. Intrinsic sugars, naturally present in unprocessed foods such as fruit and milk, which are virtually harmless. 2. Non-milk extrinsic sugars which have been removed from food's natural structure to make table sugar (sugars in cakes, confectionery, soft drinks, syrups and so on). This is the type to limit to avoid tooth decay.

---

minerals. That said, a small amount of some fats is absolutely essential for health. Strictly speaking, sugar is not needed for health, but most of us enjoy sweet things so it would be unreasonable to expect people to give up sugary food.

The problem with eating an unbalanced diet during adolescence (and earlier) is that what you eat today can contribute to tomorrow's health problems. And that doesn't just mean cases of food poisoning that follow within 6–72 hours of a meal. It means that a teenager's diet can, in part, cause or prevent heart attacks, cancer and other diseases 20 or more years on.

It may seem far-fetched to link diet during adolescence with cancer, but cancer is the second leading cause of death in the UK (heart disease is the first), and dietary factors are linked to 35% of cancer deaths. Cancer develops over many years, so just as the roots of heart disease may be traced back to childhood, so may those of cancer.

Diets that are rich in a wide variety of vegetables and fruits are associated with a reduced risk of cancer of the lung, large bowel, oesophagus and stomach. Most teenagers do not eat anywhere near enough of these fresh foods.

So this book is about helping teenagers to form eating habits that will contribute to more vitality NOW – and better long-term health.

How does YOUR diet measure up?

This is just a small selection of the food diaries filled in by teenagers as part of the research for this book. Some diets are good, but most could be improved, and several are in serious need of an overhaul. See how your diet matches up, and check out the suggestions for making easy improvements. Comments on whether teenagers are a healthy weight relate to body mass index in chapter 6.

Richard
AGE 16 · HEIGHT 1.8m (6') · WEIGHT 73.2kg (11½st)
BREAKFAST orange juice, bowl of bran flakes, piece of toast, cup of tea
LUNCH sandwiches, yogurt, apple, orange, fruit juice
EVENING MEAL pasta with tuna and prawns, peas and other vegetables; pudding: chocolate cake and ice-cream; lemonade
ACTIVITY LEVEL regular sports team member at school (cricket and rugby)

Comments
Richard is a healthy weight for his height and has a well-balanced diet. He bases meals on carbohydrate foods (good) and includes all four main food groups:
• meat and alternatives
• milk and dairy foods
• fruit and vegetables
• bread, cereals and potatoes.
Due to his age, sex, height and activity level he has high calorie needs. He seems to be meeting them as his weight is OK. However, he could eat another dairy food (milk, milk drink or yogurt) as one of his snacks each day.

Bethany
AGE 16 · HEIGHT 1.65m (5'5") · WEIGHT 62.2kg (9st 11lb)
Vegetarian
BREAKFAST orange juice, wholewheat cereal with milk and sugar,
yogurt, cup of tea
LUNCH cheese sandwiches (2 slices of wholemeal bread);
yogurt/home-made cake/chocolate bar twice a week; 1 piece of
fruit, fruit juice
AFTERNOON cereal after school, tea
EVENING MEAL pasta with vegetable sauce/jacket potato/vegetarian
casserole/macaroni cheese; chips allowed once a week; pudding:
ice-cream/pancakes/yogurt/sorbet; lemonade; tea during the
evening
ACTIVITY LEVEL 2 PE lessons of 1½ hours each per week

Comments
Bethany is a healthy weight for her height. She has a well-
balanced diet, but may need to take more care with her meat
alternatives to ensure adequate iron and zinc intake. She could eat
more iron-fortified breakfast cereals, or she could include
eggs/nuts/beans/lentils/tofu on a daily basis. For example, she
could put peanut butter or hummus in her sandwiches. She could
have beans or lentils in pasta dishes and casseroles. Wholegrain
breads and cereals are a good choice for vegetarians. Lack of iron
in Bethany's diet could lead to tiredness, poor appetite, irritability
and poor concentration. Girls' iron needs increase when
menstruation begins, and they must take special care when
becoming vegetarian.

Ben
AGE nearly 13 · HEIGHT 1.6m (5'3") · WEIGHT 45kg (7st 1lb)
Would like to put on weight and wants to build strong bones
Vegetarian

BREAKFAST 2 servings wholewheat cereal with milk and sugar, toast, fruit juice

LUNCH cheese/soft cheese wholemeal sandwiches, 1 slice home-made cake; yogurt/crisps some days; fruit juice

AFTERNOON cereal after school, squash

EVENING MEAL pasta/rice/jacket potato; chips once a week; vegetable stew/macaroni cheese/vegetarian grills or sausages once or twice a week; pudding: ice-cream/fruit/apple pie/pancakes; lemonade/squash; Complan at bedtime to help put on weight

ACTIVITY LEVEL at least 3 aerobic training sessions a week, plus football games for a professional football team's Under 16s first team; wants to be a professional footballer

Comments

Ben is a bit light for his age and height, but he has very high energy needs due to his high activity levels. These will increase again soon as he enters his growth spurt. Bone strength also greatly increases during the teenage years, so he is right to be concerned about this. Ben needs adequate vegetable protein at his lunch or evening meal on a daily basis, eg beans/lentils/Quorn/nuts/eggs /soya 'meat'. This should be eaten with large servings of starchy foods with meals, eg bread/potatoes/rice/pasta. He needs between-meal snacks, too. He could have a mid-morning snack of a sandwich/a fruit scone and a snack at supper time such as toast and milk shake/a sandwich/toasted bun or crumpet. This would replace the Complan which is not necessary. Adequate calories in a well-balanced diet is the key to fuelling growth and bone strength: 45% of bone density, or the strength of the adult skeleton, is laid down during adolescence.

Rebecca
AGE 18 · HEIGHT 1.78m (5'10") · WEIGHT 60.3kg (9st 6lb)
Previous weight was 66.3kg (10st 6lb); lost weight a few months
ago due to personal trauma, has regained half of the lost weight
and hopes to maintain present weight
Demi-vegetarian (will eat fish and chicken)
BREAKFAST not every day, but if eaten, porridge, fruit, toast/yogurt,
fruit juice and tea
MORNING chocolate bar, sometimes jelly teddies too
LUNCH cheese/cottage cheese/tuna sandwiches (2 slices of
wholemeal bread), yogurt/home-made cake, fruit juice
AFTERNOON cereal occasionally after school, tea
EVENING MEAL pasta/rice/jacket potato/pizza/fish/vegetable
stew/cauliflower grill; chips once a week; pudding: ice-
cream/yogurt/fruit; lemonade or squash; tea during the evening;
hot chocolate made with milk at bedtime
ACTIVITY LEVEL 3 aerobic sessions a week; temporarily halted
through knee injury, now having physiotherapy after knee operation

Comments
Rebecca is eating a good balance and variety of foods. Her present
weight is just about OK, but 6.3kg (1 stone) heavier would be a
healthy weight. Her lower weight of 46.3kg (8st 6lb) was definitely
too light and probably caused periods to stop. She should really have
breakfast daily, but if this is not acceptable perhaps she could have a
drink of juice and a bowl of cereal on some days. Cereal is an iron-
fortified food and good for an after-school snack. It is kinder to teeth
to have chocolate with meals rather than between meals. A banana as
a mid-morning snack would be better than confectionery

Mary
AGE 17 · HEIGHT 1.73m (5'9") · WEIGHT 60.45kg (9½st)
Went on a slimming diet of 1500-2000 calories for one month and

lost 3.15kg (½st) of which none has been regained
BREAKFAST yogurt/cereal/toast, orange juice
MORNING Club biscuit/Twix/Kit-Kat/Penguin, water
LUNCH sandwiches, fruit, yogurt, water
AFTERNOON biscuits/hot cross bun, orange squash
EVENING MEAL chicken and vegetables/pasta, orange squash;
water/orange juice/orange squash/fruit during the evening
ACTIVITY LEVEL regular exercise (aerobics, step classes, cycling,
running, rowing club)

Comments

Mary is at the low end of the healthy weight range. She did not
need to lose weight and should not lose any more, especially
considering her activity level. However, well done for not crash
dieting! Her diet is well balanced, but she should try always to eat
breakfast such as cereal and orange juice, and then have the yogurt
and some toast as optional extras. Try fruit or a scone mid
morning instead of the current chocolate and sweets which should
be eaten with meals to prevent tooth decay. Ensure some protein
(meat or alternative) filling in the lunchtime sandwiches – a good
tip for everybody. Add vegetables and/or salad and more starchy
foods (bread/potatoes/rice/pasta) to the evening meal.

Charlotte

AGE 19 · HEIGHT 1.65m (5'5") · WEIGHT 54.09kg (8½st)
BREAKFAST bowl of cereal, cup of tea
MORNING cup of tea
LUNCH 1 sandwich (2 slices of bread), cup of tea
AFTERNOON cup of coffee
EVENING MEAL meat with variety of vegetables; during the evening
600 ml (1 pint) of water; at bedtime another glass of water
ACTIVITY LEVEL at least 3 aerobic training sessions a week (county
swimmer)

Comments

Charlotte's weight is at the low end of healthy. She seems to have a
small food intake considering her activity level. If she does not eat
more she will lose weight, which will affect her swimming
performance. There is also very limited variety in her diet. Try fruit
juice with breakfast and a yogurt and fruit with lunch. Add
potato/rice/pasta/bread to the evening meal and have one or two
snacks during the day: choose from banana/yogurt/toast/fruit
scone/cereal and milk.

Jem

AGE 18 · HEIGHT 1.88m (6'2") · WEIGHT 76.36kg (12st)
BREAKFAST corn flakes and milk, orange juice, coffee
MORNING nothing to eat or drink
LUNCH meat sandwich, tea
AFTERNOON sandwich, biscuits, Wagon Wheel, orange juice
EVENING MEAL burger, carrots and potato, orange juice; during the
evening biscuits and Wagon Wheel, coffee
ACTIVITY LEVEL not much

Comments

Jem is a healthy weight for height and the balance of his diet is not
too bad, despite limited variety – he could eat more dairy foods,
fruit and vegetables. Jem could have a larger bowl of corn flakes for
breakfast. At lunch he could eat more sandwiches (some with
salad). Mid afternoon replace the biscuit or chocolate biscuit with
toast/sandwiches/cereal.

Giles

AGE 16 · HEIGHT 1.75m (5'9") · WEIGHT 70kg (11st)
When he wants to lose weight he stops eating regularly; usually
misses lunch when 'dieting'
BREAKFAST cereal/toast, milk/fruit juice/tea

MORNING tea
LUNCH sandwiches, chocolate biscuit bar, raisins, carton fruit drink
AFTERNOON milk
EVENING MEAL potatoes, peas, sausages, tomato salad, ice cream;
during the evening crisps, biscuits and tea

Comments
Giles is only a bit above average weight for his height and is not
'overweight'. If he does want to lose a few pounds, rather than skip
lunch, he could do some physical activity; he could also use semi-
skimmed milk, and replace the chocolate, crisps and ice-cream
with fruit, yogurt, fromage frais and more servings of vegetables.
Generally he could increase his intake of vegetables and fruit, and
try cereal or toast for supper instead of crisps and biscuits.

Laura
AGE 17 · HEIGHT 1.62m (5'4") · WEIGHT 57.27kg (9st)
BREAKFAST a banana, water
MORNING nothing to eat or drink
LUNCH ham sandwich, crisps, chocolate bar, water
AFTERNOON sandwiches, water
EVENING MEAL chips with chicken or other meat, peas or other
vegetable, water; during the evening biscuits and water
ACTIVITY LEVEL nil

Comments
Laura's weight is fine, but her diet is low in fruits, vegetables and
dairy foods. For breakfast she should have cereal and/or toast,
plus juice, a banana mid morning, and fruit and yogurt instead
of crisps or chocolate at lunchtime. For the evening meal reduce
the chips and try jacket potatoes/rice/pasta instead. During the
evening swap fruit or yogurt for the biscuits. What about taking
up some exercise, too for example a daily half hour walk or cycle?

Charlotte

AGE 18½ · HEIGHT 1.75m (5'9") · WEIGHT 63.63kg (10st)

Tried several diets 'off and on' but did not lose weight; also 'starves' if she wants to lose weight

Describes herself as a demi-vegetarian (occasionally eats meat, but mainly fish/poultry), faddy eater (eats only a few foods), chocoholic (1 or more chocolate bars a day) and fast-food 'addict' (2-3 takeaways a week)

BREAKFAST 2 chocolate chip cookies, a Coke, occasionally cornflakes/yogurt

MORNING chocolate/cookies/an occasional yogurt, milk/water/Coke

LUNCH (when at college) tuna sandwiches/chips; (at home) bacon sandwich/cornflakes/chicken; Coke/water

AFTERNOON yogurt/cornflakes, Coke

EVENING MEAL chicken in breadcrumbs with jacket potato and carrots/pasta/hamburger, water/milk; during the evening yogurt/cornflakes, water

ACTIVITY LEVEL does aerobics if she wants to lose weight

Comments

Charlotte is at the low end of the healthy weight range. She definitely does not need to diet but she might benefit from talking to a dietitian about changing her faddy eating habits. She may be referred to a dietitian through her family doctor. To help avoid the mid-morning chocolate attacks Charlotte could eat some cereal with milk and/or toast for breakfast, and have a yogurt mid morning and fruit (experiment to find something she likes) with lunch. Salad/vegetables/fruit with the evening meal would be good. There are several good snacks such as yogurt/milk and cereal. It would be a good idea to limit the cola drinks as they are empty calories that could harm the teeth. What about replacing some with semi-skimmed milk/milkshakes/yogurt drinks?

Stephen
AGE 18 · HEIGHT 1.78m (5'10") · WEIGHT 60.45kg (9½st)
Fast food 'addict' (takeaways 2-3 times a week)
BREAKFAST orange juice
MORNING several biscuits, coffee
LUNCH frozen lasagna/a hot dog, cup of tea
AFTERNOON nothing to eat or drink
EVENING MEAL some sort of meat dish, orange juice; during the
evening bitter or other sort of beer, peanuts/mini-cheddars/crisps,
takeaway doner kebab or ¼ pounder with cheese.
ACTIVITY LEVEL no information

Comments
Stephen is on the light side, which is not surprising considering his
eating habits. He eats little in the first part of the day and more
later on. Stephen should try cereal and toast for breakfast; adding
fruit and yogurt at lunch time; eating vegetables and a lot more
starchy foods (bread/potatoes/pasta/rice) with the evening meal.
This would help improve his diet, which is too high in fat and salt
and low in fibre. If he continues with this eating pattern he will
continue to feel tired and lethargic, and will also store up health
problems for later in life. He could have sandwiches or cereal for
supper – at least occasionally for a change.

Amy
AGE 17 · HEIGHT 1.52m (5') · WEIGHT 45.17kg (8¼st)
Vegetarian and chocoholic (one or more chocolate bars a day)
BREAKFAST orange juice, water
MORNING chocolate biscuits, hot chocolate
LUNCH sandwiches, crisps, fruit, chocolate biscuits, Ribena,
diet Coke
AFTERNOON chocolate bar, Ribena
EVENING MEAL pasta with sauce and salad/jacket potato and salad,

water; during the evening fruit/chocolate biscuits, hot orange squash/Ribena
ACTIVITY LEVEL nil

Comments

Truly a chocoholic. A very high fat and sugar intake. Amy is still in the healthy weight range, but for how long (especially with no activity)? She needs to cut back on the chocolate (yes, it is only a psychological habit, not a physical addiction). Try fruit juice, breakfast cereal and/or toast for breakfast. Have fruit or yogurt mid morning. Mid afternoon try cereal or a banana. The evening meal should include some meat alternatives such as eggs/beans/lentils/ tofu etc, plus fruit. Replace some of those sugary soft drinks between meals, too.

Christopher

AGE 17 · HEIGHT 1.83m (6') · WEIGHT 66.8kg (10½st)
Faddy eater (exists on a few limited foods)
BREAKFAST 'I don't have time for breakfast or a drink.'
MORNING hot dog
LUNCH sandwiches/soup, crisps, tea
AFTERNOON nothing to eat or drink
EVENING MEAL roast chicken/macaroni cheese/curry/chili, Robinsons Special R/orange and mango juice; during the evening toast, beer and/or vodka/Baileys
ACTIVITY LEVEL no sport or exercise

Comments

Just a healthy weight for height. Christopher shows little interest in food and is therefore unlikely to change eating habits without great motivation. What about taking up some sport or exercise? As time is important, try a quick bowl of breakfast cereal or even a milk drink for breakfast. Add some fruit at lunchtime, and vegetables and fruit to dinner (or fruit juice if that fails!). Try eating more snacks such a toast and sandwiches/cereal and milk/salad rolls and milk to drink. The main thing is to eat more vegetables, fruits and dairy foods.

Elaine

AGE 18 · HEIGHT 1.62m (5'4") · Weight 63.63kg (10st)

Has been on diets, lost about 3kg (½st) on most of them and put it all back on again; describes herself as a bit of a chocoholic, eating at least one chocolate bar a day, but does not list any chocolate in the day's eating.

BREAKFAST toast, water

MORNING nothing

LUNCH 1 round of sandwiches, occasionally crisps, water

AFTERNOON hot chocolate

EVENING MEAL usually chicken and vegetables/pasta with a meat sauce, water/milk; during the evening toast and tea

ACTIVITY LEVEL no sport or exercise

Comments

Elaine is at the top end of the healthy weight range. She is not overweight and therefore dieting will be difficult and is not necessary. Focus instead on healthier eating and increasing physical activity to stabilise, or even lose a little, weight – without really trying. Making these changes will also help get Elaine out of the slimmer's mentality (and often reduces the chocolate cravings). Eat more fruit during the day, add salad to sandwiches, and have cereal instead of toast for a change as a supper snack.

Vicky

AGE 18 · HEIGHT 1.67m (5'6") · WEIGHT 63.63kg (10st)

Demi-vegetarian and chocoholic

BREAKFAST no food, lemonade/milkshake

MORNING crisps, bread, sweets, fruit, lemonade and mineral water
LUNCH sandwiches, crisps, fruit, water
AFTERNOON water/lemonade
EVENING MEAL fish and chips/a salad, lemonade; during the
evening crisps/bread, lemonade and milkshakes
ACTIVITY LEVEL regular exercise

Comments

Vicky is within the healthy weight range; however, she's eating too
much 'junk' food. She should eat breakfast such as cereal/toast/a
fruit shake. Mid morning replace the crisps and sweets with
sandwiches and/or fruit. The evening meal should contain a good
meat alternative plus starchy foods such as bread/potatoes/
pasta/rice, plus vegetables/salad and fruit. What about trying sugar-
free lemonade to protect the teeth? And at supper time toast and
bread/cereal are preferable to the current snacks.

Sabine

AGE 18 · HEIGHT 1.62m (5'4") · WEIGHT 43.6kg (8st)
Chocoholic: says she eats about five chocolate bars a day
BREAKFAST toast or nothing, tea
MORNING chocolate
LUNCH sandwiches, chocolates, water
AFTERNOON chocolate, cakes, tea
EVENING MEAL mainly chicken/stir fries with rice, water; during
the evening chocolates, biscuits, tea
ACTIVITY LEVEL nil

Comments

Sabine is at the low end of healthy weight range and a serious
chocolate fiend, which limits her intake of vitamins and minerals
and is not good for general health or appearance – short or long-
term. Sabine does need to avoid so much chocolate as it is

replacing other healthy foods. For breakfast she should have cereal/toast plus fruit and fruit juice. Mid morning a banana, and at lunch add salad and fruit. Mid afternoon try a fruit scone/bun/milk/yogurt. In the evening meal include vegetables with the chicken and rice. For supper replace the chocolate biscuits with more cereal/toast/sandwiches/yogurt.

Sana

AGE 13 · HEIGHT 1.57m (5'2") · WEIGHT 41.36kg (6½st)

Went on one diet for 23 days; no idea of calorie content; lost 2kg (4½lb) and has not put it back on

Has decided to give up snacks between meals

BREAKFAST eggs/cereal, milk/water

MORNING nothing to eat or drink

LUNCH curry/rice, water

AFTERNOON nothing to eat or drink

EVENING MEAL (lives in Middle East and does not eat until after 10pm) curry/rice; before the meal crisps/fruit, water/orange juice, after the meal 1 biscuit and cup of tea

ACTIVITY LEVEL swimming and horse riding at least three times a week

Comments

Sana is quite underweight for her age – the ideal would be 47.72kg (7½st); she needs to gain at least 2.25kg (5lb). She should reintroduce snacks between meals and have regular meals that include a variety of meat or alternatives, rice/bread/potatoes. In addition she needs to eat more vegetables and fruits and more milk/yogurt, plus some extras such as occasional biscuits. Sana may need some help and support with her dietary changes.

Diet improving tips:

- Include breakfast on a regular basis. Choose a fortified breakfast cereal to provide iron and vitamins, plus milk for calcium. Fruit juice would be better than squash
- Add two or three pieces of fruit during the day, and a couple of servings of vegetables (in addition to potatoes)
- Try wholegrain or wholemeal bread as it contains more iron, zinc, B vitamins and fibre than white bread. This is especially important for vegetarians (but white bread is still a good food)
- Eat a wider variety of lunchtime sandwich fillings with salad or vegetables
- Have at least three servings of milk and dairy foods daily. A serving is 300ml milk, 1 small yoghurt or fromage frais, matchbox size piece of cheese.

CHAPTER 2

What teenagers are REALLY eating

There have been several recent scientific studies of teenagers' diet and lifestyle, and like the food diaries completed by teenagers for this book, these studies confirm that teenagers are eating a high fat diet and are very inactive – both risk factors for weight and health problems.

Teenagers have been brought up in an environment that discourages physical activities: with central heating, labour-saving devices and the car (or other motorised transport). Teenagers (like most of us) no longer have to help with heavy physical work at home or work, and they simply do not run, walk or cycle any more. Leisure pastimes are inactive: 'flaking out', sleeping and watching tv. The average person in Britain now watches 26 hours of tv a week (compared to 13 hours in the 1960s), and the average British school pupil watches three hours of tv a day. As one prominent American doctor (Dr William Dietz of Boston Harvard Medical School) puts it: 'tv or not tv, fat is the question …'

Not only is the teenage diet high in fat, but it is also low in vitamins and minerals, so young people are running on poor-quality fuel. This leaves them feeling lethargic. Further, anyone with a genetic predisposition to weight gain who has that sort of lifestyle will, in time, have weight problems and eventually may become obese. Like the rest of society, there are going to be more unfit and overweight teenagers than would occur if just a small amount of exercise were taken and better quality (more nutrient-dense) foods were eaten.

The habit of skipping meals and snacking on confectionery and crisps also means teenagers are not feeding their brains well throughout the day. This may worsen mood swings (which are naturally up and down during adolescence) and impair academic achievement – especially under stress conditions such as exams – and overall memory.

The pessimistic view – more heart attacks at a younger age

The typical teenage diet is precisely what experts would expect from a country with one of the highest incidences of heart disease in the world. Diets both at home and at school are bad – it is hard to say which is worse as they are often both so poor. One of the only things that can be said with certainty is that if teenagers continue to eat the same sort of food when they become adults, it can pretty confidently be predicted that the UK will continue to have one of the highest heart disease rates in the world. The heart attack rate may even go up and the age of victims come down.

The optimistic view – they will grow out of it

If adolescent eating habits are 'rebellious' and 'experimental', then the current high fat intake should reduce as adolescents become adults and modify their eating habits. This will reduce risks to health and cure weight problems. Similarly high sugar intake from soft drinks, confectionery and sugar should decline with age.

What are 15- to 25-year-olds eating?

One of the most comprehensive surveys of the dietary habits of young people (1,000 15- to 25-year-olds) showed average fat intake of both boys and girls to be 43% of energy (it should ideally be no more than 35% total fat and no more than 11% saturated fat).

- Both boys and girls had lower than recommended iron intakes.
- Girls in their late teens, who described themselves as diet-conscious, had low iron intakes, risking, in particular, anaemia and tiredness.
- Average riboflavin (vitamin B2) intake was lower than recommended.

Women and men in their late teens who live alone are especially likely to eat too little with consequential low intakes of some B vitamins. Teenage males have low intakes of B vitamins (thiamin, nicotinic acid, B12 and folic acid). Women in their late teens have the lowest and least adequate of all nutrient intakes. Particularly low were calcium, thiamin, riboflavin, folic acid and vitamin C and iron. This would be of real concern in teenage pregnancies (see pages 90-92).

Those aged 15 to 18 years did marginally better on nutrient intake, but intakes of iron were still low and they were still eating fewer calories than needed for normal growth, yet as growth seemed OK, they were probably very inactive.

Women in all age groups who considered themselves to be overweight or who were watching their diet had the least satisfactory intakes.

All those surveyed were asked to list foods they liked but should not eat. The most frequently mentioned foods, in order of popularity, were chocolate, chips, sweets and toffees, cakes and buns, fried fatty foods, crisps and cream cakes. When asked why they felt they should not eat so much of these foods, the main reason given was because they were fattening. Few teenagers mentioned soft or fizzy drinks as undesirable or fattening (most contained sugar then, rather than artificial sweeteners), despite 39% of 15- to 18-year-olds consuming them on a daily basis.

- 39% of 15- to 18-year-olds ate sweets on a daily basis
- 39% said they drank alcohol between one and three times a week

- 68% of 19-year-olds drank alcohol at least once a week
- 8% ate sausages or meat pies every day, and 64% ate them one to three times a week
- 22% ate ketchup and sauce on a daily basis

Breakfast

Fifteen peer cent of 15- to 18-year-olds and 19% of 19- to 21-year-olds never ate breakfast, rising to 28% of those who always watched what they ate.

What are schoolchildren eating?

A survey of more than 3,000 10- to 11-year-olds and 14- to 15-year-olds showed that around one quarter of British schoolchildren consume more than 40% of their calories in the form of fats. About half the children had intakes of 35–40% of energy provided by fat.

- 14- and 15-year-old girls were eating less iron than the recommended amounts.
- Older girls on slimming diets were particularly likely to have low iron intakes. They were also eating less riboflavin (vitamin B2) than they needed because they were consuming less breakfast cereal (many of which are fortified with this vitamin) and milk – probably because they were skipping breakfast.
- 60% of older girls were consuming less calcium than recommended, probably because they were drinking little milk and eating little bread and other cereals.
- Among children eating too little fresh vegetables and fruit there were low intakes of beta-carotene.
- There was also concern that vitamin D intake was not enough for rapid growth and bone development during teen years.

School meals – too fatty by far

The survey also looked at school meals. Since the abolition of Nutritional Standards for school meals in 1980, these no longer have to provide one third of children's vitamins and minerals and 40% of protein. The survey used the previously prescribed nutritional standards as desirable for school meals and thought it reasonable that a school meal should provide one third of a child's daily energy intake. The biggest criticism of school meals was that they provided more than 40% of calories as fat. It was recommended that the fat (as chips, fried foods, pastry products) should be replaced by starchy foods such as pasta, bread, potatoes (other than chips or crisps) and fruit and vegetables. This would also improve vitamin and mineral intake.

What you can do to improve school meals

An excellent way of finding out how healthy the school meals are at any school with which you are associated is to use the School Meals Assessment Pack (SMAP). It contains an easy-to-use computer programme which tells you how the average school meal served scores against nutritional guidelines. It can also indicate whether the food that an individual pupil chooses over a week meets the nutritional guidelines. The pack can be used by parents, governors or senior pupils in Home Economics or Information Technology lessons to analyse their school menu and devise and improve menus to meet nutritional guidelines. With pupil involvement changes will be better received.

For more information about how to agree a policy on healthy food at school, how to market school meals, the ins and outs of catering contracts, how to get organised and get others involved see booklets from The School Meals Campaign, PO Box 402, London WC1H 9TZ, telephone 0171 383 7638. The School Meals Assessment Pack (£40) is available from The School Meals Campaign (above). It was compiled by the National Heart Forum in partnership with British Heart Foundation, The British Diabetic Association and Camden & Islington Community Health Services NHS Trust.

Other lunchtime meals – just as bad

The children who ate out of school at cafés and fast food outlets had lower than average daily intakes of some vitamins and minerals, and these were not made up by the foods eaten at other times of the day and at home. Iron intakes of older girls were particularly affected, and they also ate less protein, B vitamins, calcium and vitamin D than other pupils. Generally the nutritional quality of the diets of children eating out at cafés was even poorer than the sometimes nutritionally inadequate school meals. Children who went home for lunch fared better.

What are 16- and 17-year-olds eating?

A study of more than 4,500 16- and 17-year-olds revealed diets too high in fat and sugar and too low in starchy foods that contain natural fibre.

- Average fat intake was 42% of total energy (more than the 35% maximum recommended). The main sources of fat in these teenagers' diets were meat and meat products including pies, burgers, sausages and kebabs (23%), fats and oils (18%), fried potatoes (13%), cereals and cereal products (18%) and milk and milk products (12%).
- Average sugar intake was 13% of calories (more than the recommended maximum of 10%).
- Average intake of fibre was 15g per day (less than the recommended 18g per day).
- Only 25% of boys and 10% of girls in the study met fibre targets of 18g per day set for adults. The main sources of fibre were chips and breakfast cereals. Better sources than chips would be fibre in beans, oats, vegetables and fruit which are also less 'fattening' than chips.
- Average intakes of iron, magnesium and folates were below recommended levels. Low intakes of green vegetables among

teenage girls are related to a lack of magnesium and folates.

- Nearly half of the boys and girls had drunk alcohol during the four days of the food diary. The amounts drunk were within low risk levels. However, researchers say teenagers are notoriously inaccurate with reporting alcohol intake (lowering actual level if parental disapproval is likely, or exaggerating the amount drunk in circumstances where it is considered more 'adult' to drink more).

16- and 17-year-old female slimmers

Of those girls from the above study who were slimming, twice as many failed to achieve RNIs (recommended nutrient intakes, the amount thought to cover everyone's needs; see also chapter 4) for thiamin, riboflavin, folates, B12, B6, zinc, copper and selenium. Predictably they ate more foods associated with dieting such as low-fat spread, skimmed milk, cottage cheese, yogurt, salad vegetables, fruit and fruit juice. Yet even so they still obtained 40.5% of their total calories from fat (more than the 35% recommended, and only slightly less than their non-slimming peers who ate 42.5% calories as fat). They still ate a lot of sugary foods – the same amounts as the non-dieters. To improve their vitamin and mineral intakes they could have included more nutrient-dense foods in their diets, such as fortified breakfast cereals and low-fat diary products.

Lunchtime food of 11- and 12-year-olds outside the home

A survey in 1992 found that school meals contributed more than half the calories of this age group outside the home. Nutritional analysis showed the school meals to be high in fat (mainly from chips), supplying 43% of energy from fats, and vitamin C (fruit juice). However, school meals provided less sugar and more protein, calcium, iron and vitamin C than packed lunches, home lunches (same fat content as school meals, so parents did no better), shops and takeaways. Lunches bought from shops and takeaways were lowest in protein, calcium and iron and highest in sugar.

Which? way to improve school meals

When *Which?*, the Consumers' Association magazine, looked at school meals in 1992 (12 years after nutritional standards for school meals were abolished, removing any requirement for schools to provide a well-balanced school meal), they found the food on sale in cash cafeterias to be very similar to that on sale in the schools' local chip shops, takeaways and 'greasy spoon' cafés.

Most of the 14- and 15-year-olds in the survey chose the fattier snack foods, and many chose just chips and a fizzy drink for lunch, having spent most of their money earlier in the day on confectionery, crisps and other fizzy drinks. The lunches in the food diaries studied were high in fat and sugar, and low in fibre, iron and folates.

The packed lunches taken to school by the children in the *Which?* survey typically contained sandwiches, a packet of crisps, a chocolate bar and a sweet soft drink. Only one in four took fruit. Crisps, chocolate, chips, biscuits (chocolate coated) and sweet drinks from vending machines in the schools – none supplied fruit or fruit juice – supplemented packed and school lunches.

Although the above studies show that many teenage girls are not meeting recommended daily intakes of iron and riboflavin, and girls on slimming diets may be failing to meet recommendations for a wider number of nutrients, they may not be deficient because the recommended amounts include a safety margin. However, if these patterns of eating continue they could, over time, harm health. And none will be in a state of 'optimum health'.

What surveys and opinion polls say teenagers are eating

From time to time 'vox pop' surveys and polls purport to tell us the nation's habits and attitudes. Usually these have a vested commercial interest and the statistics may be interpreted to suit the aims of individuals and companies who are trying to sell us something.

However, the bare statistics from these surveys are interesting.

Skipping breakfast, snacking, eating takeaways

A survey of 1,000 British adults (Del Monte Extra Healthy Lifestyle Report, commissioned for the launch of Extra fruit juice with added vitamins) claimed that 16- to 24-year-olds have the unhealthiest diet of any age group of the population. The claim was made on the basis of questions about the popularity of breakfast, fast foods and snacks, whether the interviewees thought they were overweight, how many colds they got, whether they thought (Del Monte) fruit juice would prevent colds and flu, and so on ... Of the 16- to 24-year-old group surveyed:

- 16% never ate breakfast
- 58% ate fast food takeaways once a week or more, 29% ate them two to three times a week
- 78% regularly ate snacks between meals.

The same survey asked whether people's eating habits had changed during the last five years. Again, looking at 16- to 24-year-olds within the survey:

- 28% claimed to eat more fried foods than five years ago
- 20% ate less fresh fruit.
  Of most concern from the survey is that:
- 5% of children (under 16 years old) ate breakfast only once a week or even less frequently
- 18% of parents thought their children's diet less healthy than their diet as children
- 30% of parents believed their children's diet did not contain enough vitamins for good health

In the same survey, in 13% of homes a family meal took place only once a week or less often. To counter this, 82% of respondents in the north east and 56% in the south did eat a family meal together on a daily basis.

Snackaholic teenagers too busy to eat

A survey of 1,000 women aged 16-24 (conducted for Boots during the winter of 1994) found this age group twice as likely to skip breakfast as any other age group. In addition:

- 50% of women aged 16-24 were too busy to eat a balanced diet
- 42% were too busy to have proper meals regularly, finding it more convenient to snack or miss meals
- 33% ate crisps and chocolates at lunchtime instead of lunch
- 33% ate an unbalanced evening meal

Busy lifestyle puts teenage health at risk

Another survey by Boots of 1,016 adults (aged over 12), carried out during January 1996, shows that things have not improved much in two years. Of the 15- to 24-year-old age group in the survey, nearly a quarter said they missed meals when they were busy (at work or college or school); 60% grabbed a snack when and where they could in the same circumstances; and less than a quarter made time to eat a meal (compared with half in the 25- to 34-year-old group and more in the 45- to 50-year-old group).

The typical meal pattern among 15- to 24-year-olds revealed in the survey was:

BREAKFAST – a quick coffee (although 30% had nothing at all) and maybe a chocolate bar on the way to school or work
LUNCH – typically a sandwich, a chocolate bar and a soft drink
EVENING –the only meal of the day

Nearly half of 15- to 24-year-olds said this left them feeling anything from unwell to under the weather, yet they did not do anything to improve their eating habits and so improve the way they felt.

In addition, only a quarter of 15- to 24-year-olds regularly found time to unwind and relax during the evening – 40% watched tv, 30% 'flaked out' by the evening, 20% fell asleep. Only 13% took regular exercise as a way of relaxing.

Chips, crisps, chocolate and Cola

Good Housekeeping magazine asked 200 children aged 11-14 to keep a diary of everything they ate and drank, and then analysed the diets to assess nutritional value. They found the results 'disturbing':

- almost 8 out of 10 children failed to eat enough calcium
- 9 out of 10 ate too little iron
- 7 out of 10 ate more than the recommended level of fat
- nearly half ate chips or crisps at least twice a day
- only 1 in 100 ate the target figure of five portions of fruit and vegetables a day
- 56% ate no fruit and vegetables at all

One child's lunchbox in the survey contained a can of cola, a can of fizzy orange drink, a packet of roast chicken flavoured crisps, a packet of prawn cocktail crisps and a kingsize Mars bar.

'Impossible' to swap apples for chocolate

According to a survey of 11,000 people carried out for the Co-op, the real diet of the nation is very different from the role model of healthy eating, the National Plate Guide (page 46). It adds up to:

bread, other cereal and potatoes – 21%

fruit and vegetables – 24%

meat, fish and alternatives – 18%

milk and dairy foods – 19%

fatty and sugary foods – 18%

This means that many families are eating twice as much fatty and sugary food as they should and far too little starchy foods, fruits and vegetables. Most disturbingly, the Co-op survey suggests that 11- to 16-year-olds are eating three times as much fatty and sugary food as they should. Nearly one third of their diet is fatty and sugary food.

The reasons for not eating more healthily vary. Those who had got the messages about healthy eating did not put their knowledge into practice because they felt it would take too long, cost too much and be too much hassle. They felt they needed help to put it into action. Others were not convinced that healthy eating matters. The majority got their diet advice from the media and found conflicting stories confusing, so they did not act.

Speed, convenience and simplicity were the priorities of most consumers who claimed no time to plan ahead for meals and shopping trips; instead they ate what came to hand. Parents said it was not possible to convince children to eat an apple rather than a bar of chocolate. The conclusion of the study was that most people were unlikely to eat more healthily – unless a major event such as a heart attack or pregnancy intervened.

A question of balance
A questionnaire on teenage eating habits by the National Dairy Council was completed by 1,302 children aged 11 to 16 years. Analysis revealed meal skipping, poorly balanced diets, high intakes of sugary and fatty drinks and foods, and low intakes of iron-rich and calcium-rich foods.

Half the teenagers thought they ate a balanced diet, yet most ate fewer than four daily servings of starchy food or fruit and vegetables, and 16% ate no vegetables or fresh fruit (9%).

Half also ate high fat/sugar snacks (biscuits, cakes, chocolate, puddings, sweets, crisps and other savoury snacks) at least four times a day – far more than the ideal. And 10% ate these snacks ten or more times a day. In addition:
- 22% skip breakfast.
- 95% snack between meals – 20% on the way to school, 57% mid-morning, 19% on the way home, 69% after school, 46% during the evening and 53% before bed.
- Crisps were the most popular snack, followed by chocolates and sweets, cakes and biscuits.

CHAPTER 3

How to improve what teenagers are eating

It's all very well to be told that you get all the nutrients (vitamins and minerals) you need if you eat a well-balanced diet. But what is a well-balanced diet?

Fruit and vegetables
Choose a wide variety

Bread, other cereals and potatoes
Eat all types and choose high fibre kinds whenever you can

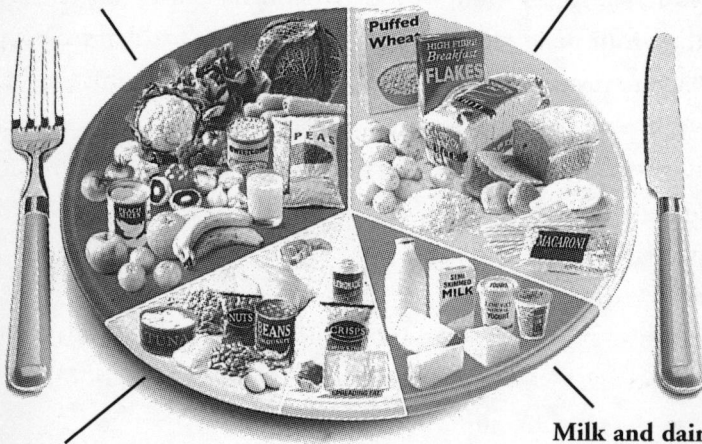

Meat, fish and alternatives
Choose lower fat alternatives whenever you can

Fatty and sugary foods
Try not to eat these too often, and when you do, have small amounts

Milk and dairy foods
Choose lower fat alternati whenever you can

Source: The National Food Guide, reproduced with permission from the Health Education Authority.

The plate model illustrates the proportion of foods on the plate that make up a well-balanced meal, and a well-balanced diet. There are four food groups that contribute to health and vitality. The group that we could do with the least, and which most teenagers eat too much of, is the fatty and sugary food group.

The main nutrients from the food groups in the healthy eating plate model are: Bread, other cereals and potatoes – B vitamins, calcium, iron; Fruits and vegetables – vitamin C, beta carotene, folates, magnesium; Milk and dairy foods – vitamins A, D, B12, calcium; Meat, fish and alternatives – B vitamins, iron, magnesium, zinc.

Teen-ie steps in the right direction

Many teenagers' diets are a long way from the ideal. The following are the first steps in the right direction.

1 Make better choices of snacks – see the 28 Day Healthy Eating Plan and Good Snack Guide chapters for inspiration.

2 Do not skip meals – you will miss out on all the nutrients you need, and be tempted to eat even more poor quality snacks.

3 Eat sugary foods (a limited number) at meals and not between meals, to reduce tooth decay.

4 Boost intake of foods rich in nutrients that may be missing from your diet. You will have gained a good idea of the weak spots in your eating patterns from the teenage diaries and the studies reported in the previous chapter.

The charts that follow give a more detailed picture of how to build a well balanced diet.

WOMEN	Bread, potatoes, pasta and other cereals	Vegetables and fruit
	These foods should be the main part of most meals. An example of a portion is a slice of bread or a medium potato, or 2 tbsp cooked rice/pasta or a bowl of breakfast cereal.	Eat a mixture of different types. An example of a portion is a medium banana or an apple, a glass of juice, a side salad, 3 tbsp vegetables (cooked from fresh, frozen, canned).
11–14 Active	These foods provide you with the energy you need to grow and be active. They should be the main part of most meals and snacks. Eat about 7–9 portions a day.	Aim for at least 5 portions a day.
11–14 Sedentary	Eat about 5–7 portions a day.	
15–18 Active	Eat about 9-11 portions a day.	
15–18 Sedentary	Eat about 7-9 portions a day.	
19+ Active	Eat about 8-10 portions a day.	
19+ Sedentary	Eat about 6-8 portions a day.	

Milk and dairy foods	Meat, fish and alternatives	Fats and fatty and sugary foods
Choose lower fat versions whenever you can. An example of a portion is a glass of milk, a small pot of yogurt or a matchbox size piece of cheese.	Eat fish, especially oily fish, at least twice a week. Remove fat from meat or buy low-fat types. An example of a portion is a chicken breast, a medium fillet of fish, or 3 tbsp of cooked beans, peas or lentils.	Use low-fat monounsaturated or polyunsaturated spreads. For cooking use small amounts of polyunsaturated or monounsaturated oils.
Eat about 3 portions a day. Calcium is particularly important in building and maintaining bones.	Eat about 2 portions a day. Vegetarians can obtain iron to prevent anaemia from foods like lentils and peas. Iron is absorbed better if fruits and vegetables containing vitamin C are eaten at the same time.	If you are active one or two sugary or fatty foods a day (e.g cream, cakes, pastries, savoury snacks, fried foods), will do no harm as part of a balanced diet. Eat sugary foods and drinks with meals to reduce tooth decay.
	Eat about 2-3 portions a day.	
Eat about 2-3 portions a day.	Eat about 2 portions a day.	

MEN	Bread, potatoes, pasta and other cereals	Vegetables and fruit
	These foods should be the main part of most meals. An example of a portion is a slice of bread or a medium potato, or 2 tbsp cooked rice/pasta or a bowl of breakfast cereal.	Eat a mixture of different types. An example of a portion is a medium banana or an apple, a glass of juice, a side salad, 3 tbsp vegetables (cooked from fresh, frozen, canned).
11–14 Active	These foods provide you with the energy you need to grow and be active. They should be the main part of most meals and snacks, eat about 9-11 portions a day.	Aim for at least 5 portions a day, more is fine.
11–14 Sedentary	Eat about 7–9 portions a day.	
15–18 Active	You have very high energy needs at this stage in your life. These foods provide you with the energy you need to grow and be active. They should be the main part of most meals and snacks. Eat about 11–14 portions a day.	
15–18 Sedentary	Eat about 9-10 portions a day.	
19+ Active	Eat about 10-11 portions a day.	
19+ Sedentary	Eat about 9–10 portions a day.	

Milk and dairy foods	Meat, fish and alternatives	Fats and fatty and sugary foods
Choose lower fat versions whenever you can. An example of a portion is a glass of milk, a small pot of yogurt or a matchbox size piece of cheese.	Eat fish, especially oily fish, at least twice a week. Remove fat from meat or buy low-fat types. An example of a portion is a chicken breast, a medium fillet of fish, or 3 tbsp of cooked beans, peas or lentils.	Use low-fat monounsaturated or polyunsaturated spreads. For cooking use small amounts of polyunsaturated or monounsaturated oils.
Eat about 3 portions a day.	Eat about 2-3 portions a day . Vegetarians can obtain iron to prevent anaemia from foods such as beans, lentils and peas. Iron is absorbed better if fruits and vegetables containing vitamin C are eaten at the same time.	If you are active one or two sugary or fatty foods a day (e.g cream, cakes, pastries, savoury snacks, fried foods), will do no harm as part of a balanced diet. Eat sugary foods and drinks with meals to reduce tooth decay.
	Eat about 3 portions a day.	
Eat about 2-3 portions a day.	Eat about 2-3 portions a day.	
Eat about 2 portions a day.		

Should I take vitamin supplements?

Balancing the diet as in the plate guide and tables should provide enough vitamins and minerals, but the reality is that many teenagers' diets are far from ideal:

- Many teenagers rely on a few foods and might be described as faddy eaters.
- Many teenagers eat a large proportion of so-called junk food or processed foods that are high in fat and sugar.
- Girls in particular eat restricted slimming diets.
- Hardly any teenagers eat enough vegetables and fruits.

All this, coupled with the fact that teenagers are eating fewer calories than they did a generation ago, and not eating enough nutrient rich foods, means that they are likely also to be short of vitamins and minerals. These patterns of eating are not advisable for any age group and are especially risky during the teens when there is a period of rapid growth that increases the demands for calories, vitamins and minerals. Intakes of iron, calcium in particular and many other vitamins and minerals have fallen in this generation of teenagers.

Vitamins and Minerals

Vitamins are substances needed in small amounts for growth and normal daily body chemistry. It is essential to eat vitamins in food because the body cannot make them (with the exception of vitamin D, which is made by the action of sunlight on the skin, and vitamins B12 and K2 made by intestinal bacteria).

Minerals are substances needed for normal function of the body, for example in enzymes. Trace elements and minerals are required in minute amounts.

Minimum cooking and preparation protects vitamins

Cooking doesn't destroy minerals, but it does allow them to leach out into cooking water, so use the liquid in soups and sauces.

Vitamin pill warning

If dietary supplements are taken it is important that they are taken in balance because vitamins and minerals work together in the body. Too much of any one particular nutrient might be toxic or unbalance the system and be as detrimental in some ways as not having enough. Supplements cannot be taken in place of food.

It is not known whether pills are as beneficial as vitamin-rich foods, which contain other substances such as the antioxidant flavonoids and carotenoids that may work with vitamins and minerals to help prevent heart disease and cancer and maintain health. Similarly, a diet rich in starchy, naturally high-fibre foods (bread, pasta, rice, beans, potatoes), vegetables and fruits keeps the digestive system healthy, aids weight control and protects against cancer, heart disease and so on – which pills probably cannot do.

Antioxidant protection

Protecting body cells from damage caused by free radicals is very important in maintaining good health. Antioxidant nutrients work together in the body so it is important that we obtain enough of each. The main antioxidants are vitamins C, E and beta-carotene, and the minerals zinc, copper, selenium and manganese. Some antioxidants such as vitamin E are difficult to obtain from even a well-planned diet. The best sources include vegetables and fruits – which teenagers eat irregularly – and vegetable oils. Vegetarian women usually have a high intake of antioxidants because they eat more vegetables and fruits but other groups may benefit from supplementation with antioxidant nutrients.

Nutrients at risk in a teenage diet

Calcium

Eating too little calcium increases the risk of osteoporosis. Adolescent girls increasing their dairy food intake have, in one study, gained 7% bone mineral density over a year.

GOOD SOURCES OF ANTIOXIDANT NUTRIENTS

MINERALS	FOOD SOURCES
Zinc	Meat, milk and milk products, bread, cereals, cereal products, especially wholegrain, eggs, shellfish
Manganese	Wholegrain cereals, nuts, tea
Selenium	Cereals, especially bread, fish, liver, pork, cheese, eggs, walnuts, brazil nuts
Copper	Wholegrain cereals, meat, vegetables, dried fruit, nuts, pulses, liver
VITAMINS	FOOD SOURCES
Beta carotene	Yellow and orange fruits and vegetables, particularly: carrots, broccoli, tomatoes, melons, apricots, peaches, pumpkin, watercress
Vitamin C	Fruit and vegetables, particularly: citrus fruit, blackcurrants, strawberries, kiwi fruit, gooseberries, guava, green leafy vegetables, green peppers, swede, parsnips
Vitamin E	Vegetable oils, particularly sunflower seed oils, almonds, hazelnuts, wholegrain breakfast cereals, wholemeal bread, dark green vegetables, wheatgerm. The best fruit and vegetable sources are: apples, bananas, blackcurrants, damsons. Vegetables: asparagus, broccoli, carrots, peas, spinach, parsley, tomatoes, lettuce, watercress
Vitamin A	Liver, kidneys, full-fat dairy products, oily fish, fortified margarine NB Beta-carotene from plant foods can also be turned into vitamin A in the body

Source: The Ultimate ACE Diet, Janette Marshall, Vermilion

Half of all British schoolgirls have experimented with slimming diets, and the National Osteoporosis Society estimates that they could be at risk of fractured bones from osteoporosis as early as their thirties: low calorie and low calcium intakes weaken bones at a critical time of development.

Osteoporosis literally means 'porous bone'. Loss of bone mass happens in everyone around age 35, but in osteoporosis it goes so far that it causes bones to be likely to fracture. A fall, blow or lifting action that would not normally be a problem can easily break a bone in someone with osteoporosis. Osteoporosis results in more than 150,000 fractures (typically hip fractures) each year.

Although osteoporosis does not usually affect women until their sixties, prevention should start young. Studies show that the more milk drunk before age 25 the less likely is osteoporosis. Most calcium is accumulated in the bones during the teens, so calcium intake needs to be high then.

Even once bones have stopped growing they continue to rebuild themselves and lose calcium, for example during pregnancy when the growing baby demands calcium, or when taking certain medicines. Hormone levels also affect calcium, and calcium losses occur with the loss of oestrogen production at the menopause. HRT (hormone replacement therapy) reduces the risk of osteoporosis.

Best food sources of calcium: Dairy foods provide 58% of calcium in the British diet. Calcium in milk is the most easily used by the body. The naturally occurring lactose (milk sugars) and casein (protein) aid absorption. Calcium from soya products is also well absorbed.

Choose: low-fat milk, cheese and yogurt, tofu (made using calcium compound, check labels), leafy green vegetables, canned fish such as sardines/pilchards and whitebait (because the bones are eaten), soya milk fortified with calcium. Vegetarians obtain more of their calcium from sesame seeds, tahini and eggs.

Are you getting enough calcium?

This table shows typical sources of calcium in the diet with approximate amounts in common portion sizes given as calcium units (1 unit = 50mg calcium). To estimate daily intake, multiply the portions of food consumed by the number of calcium units, and then add all the values together. For example, one portion of cheese plus two slices of bread would give: 6 + 1 = 7 calcium units.

DAILY CALCIUM CALCULATOR			
FOOD SOURCE	Calcium Units	Portions Eaten	Calcium Units Consumed
Hard cheese (40g of cheddar)	6		
Milk (200ml)	5		
Low-fat natural yogurt (125g pot)	5		
Canned pilchards, or other canned fish (45g)	3		
Tofu (100g)	3		
Spinach, cooked (90g)	3		
Broccoli spears, cooked (60g)	½		
Canned beans or peas, cooked (90g)	½		
Watercress (30g)	1		
Carrots, cooked (60g)	⅓		
Egg, hard boiled (1 large)	½		
Bread, white (1 slice)	½		
Target: Girls 16 units (800mg) Boys 20 units (1000mg) Parents 14 units (700 mg)	Daily total of calcium units eaten		

Source: Boots and National Osteoporosis Society

Magnesium

Magnesium is another essential mineral for healthy bones. It works with calcium to regulate the body's metabolism and is needed for the body to convert food (calories) into energy.

Best food sources of magnesium: soya beans, nuts, wholemeal flour and bread, cereals, peas, dried fruit, green vegetables, peanuts. Chocolate also contains magnesium, but you should only be eating it as a treat! Overdose of magnesium is unlikely because an intake higher than 2g per day passes through the intestine unabsorbed. However too much could interfere with absorption of other minerals and harm people susceptible to kidney stones.

Phosphorus

Phosphorus is needed for bone strength and may be lacking, or in poor ratio to calcium if dairy food intake is low or lots of fizzy drinks are taken. It is widely available from a balanced diet.

Vitamin D

Vitamin D is also necessary for strong bones because it enables the skeleton to absorb calcium. Vitamin D is found in butter, margarine, oily fish and other fats and oily fish. It is called the sunlight vitamin, because it is made by the action of sunlight (not sunbathing) on the skin. Sitting by an open window with bare hands and face for about 20 minutes a day should be enough for housebound people.

Very rarely teenagers might need supplementary vitamin D if the diet does not include it and the skin is very dark or not exposed to natural daylight because of clothing or an indoor lifestyle.

B vitamins

Stress from juggling the demands of school, college, work and family may evoke the body's stress response, increasing the need for vitamin C and the B vitamins, riboflavin, thiamin and vitamin B6.

Folic acid – a special need

Folic acid is another B vitamin. Low intakes have been linked to an increased risk of babies being born with spina bifida and related conditions. The greatest protection is afforded when folic acid supplements are taken from the time a woman begins trying to conceive until the twelfth week of pregnancy. This differs from the traditional approach, where attention is focused on regular ante-natal care, sometimes starting after the first two or three months of pregnancy. It is now known that pre-pregnancy nutrition is vital, so attention is switching to ensure good diet before conception as well as through pregnancy.

In addition to taking folic acid supplements, before conception or as pregnancy is suspected (for example, if there is a risk of pregnancy following unprotected sexual intercourse), foods rich in folic acid (folates) should also be eaten – and not overcooked as heat destroys the vitamin. There is no danger of taking in more than the recommended dosage (see below) because folic acid is a water-soluble B vitamin and any excess will be lost in the urine without any harm to the body – or baby. See also teenage pregnancy guidelines pages 90-92. Good food sources of folic acid include: brussels sprouts, asparagus, spinach, kale, black eye beans, fortified breads and breakfast cereals, broccoli, spring greens, cabbage, green beans, cauliflower, peas and cooked soya beans.)

Folic acid tablets for women

Don't be confused about the terms 'folate' and 'folic acid'. Folates are derived from folic acid and the form which occurs naturally in foods. Folic acid is the form in which this particular type of B vitamin is taken as vitamin supplements. All sexually active women should be aware of the need for folic acid supplements at 0.4mg or 400mcg daily. They are available on prescription, but unless you qualify for free prescriptions, they are cheaper to buy from the chemist.

Quiz: Are you getting enough iron?

1 Do you eat any meat, fish or poultry (or foods containing them, such as meat or fish pies) at least three times a week
Yes (score 4)   **No (score 0)**

2 Do you drink three or more glasses of red wine, on average, each week?
Yes (score 2)   **No (score 0)**

3 Do you drink fruit juice or eat citrus fruit with meals at least three times a week?
Yes (score 3)   **No (score 0)**

4 Do you sprinkle raw bran on breakfast cereals or other foods?
Yes (score 0)   **No (score 3)**

5 Do you usually drink tea or coffee with or immediately after your main meals?
Yes (score 0)   **No (score 3)**

6 Do you eat very little or, from time to time, go on low-calorie (slimming) diets?
Yes (score 0)   **No (score 3)**

7 Do you go marathon running or regularly take heavy exercise?
Yes (score 0)   **No (score 1)**

8 Women only: do you usually have moderate or heavy periods?
Yes (score 0)   **No (score 4)**

Scoring: Add up your score for each question. If you regularly take iron tablets or tonics, or vitamin pills containing iron, add 3 points.
Men 0-6 Women 0-15 You may well be short of iron. You need to eat more iron-rich foods, eat fruit after meals and drink juice with meals instead of tea or coffee.
Men 7-16 Women 16-20 You are probably getting enough iron. If you take supplements see if you can increase your iron intake from food instead.
Men 17-21 Women 21-25 You are getting enough iron. If you're taking a supplement you could probably do without it.

Period problems and dietary supplements

Many teenage girls and women suffer from PMS (premenstrual syndrome). They are prone to mood swings, irritability, bloating, craving foods such as chocolate, and other symptoms before a period. Some doctors say there is no link between eating and period problems. Others think a change in diet – especially eating little and often eg three small meals and three small snacks daily, with minimal sugar – or a vitamin supplement, might be useful.

The first line of defence is to eat a well-balanced diet and replace some coffee, tea and cola with decaffeinated versions or non-caffeine drinks. However, if vitamin pills or other dietary supplements are taken to alleviate symptoms of PMS, make notes over three months (or three cycles) to see if there is a noticeable benefit. One single treatment may not solve period problems. The answer may lie in a combination, such as a change of diet and one or two supplements, plus exercise and relaxation techniques to remove tension.

Low intakes of certain vitamins and minerals have been linked to PMS. While properly conducted scientific trials do not show much benefit from taking vitamins, vitamin B6 is prescribed and self-prescribed for treatment of PMS. Stick to the recommended dosages because B6 can be harmful if more than 100mg is taken daily – even though it is a water-soluble vitamin. Other nutrients that might help are vitamin C, vitamin E, magnesium and calcium. Magnesium may be low in the diets of women, and one trial claims to have shown a reduction in anxiety and irritability among women taking a magnesium supplement.

Several trials have also shown evening primrose oil to reduce PMS symptoms in some women. The oil contains a particular type of polyunsaturated fatty acid, gamma-linolenic acid (GLA), which is used by the body to make prostaglandins. These hormone-like substances regulate the effects of hormones controlling the menstrual cycle. They are also involved in other chemical reactions. Breast tenderness seems to respond well to evening primrose oil, and many women have reported other improvements, although it does not work for all women. GLA is also found in borage oil and blackcurrant seed oil and can also be formed from linoleic acid in vegetable oils (eg sunflower, corn, safflower). Vitamin E is linked to prostaglandin metabolism; it is not so easy to get large amounts from food, but try vegetable oils, fortified spreads/margarines and nuts.

Vitamins and the pill
Women taking the contraceptive pill have lower levels of vitamin B6 in their bloodstream. While they are apparently healthy, there may be some benefit in taking vitamin B6 supplements. Good food sources of B6 are wheatgerm (wholemeal breads and Hovis contain it), oats, liver, soya flour, bananas, nuts and yeast extract. See the overdose warning above.

The time of your life
If vitamin and mineral supplements are taken, it is better, in many instances, to choose a formula that has been designed for a particular time of life (eg menstruation, pregnancy) or for particular lifestyles (eg for vegetarians, teenagers, busy people who do not eat a balanced diet). A dietary supplement needs to be taken for a minimum of three months to receive full benefit.

Popping vitamin pills does not preclude the need for a well-balanced diet.

Vitamin pills and IQ

Improvements in academic test scores (and pupil behaviour) were reported from America after changes were made in the school meals provided for 800,000 New York school pupils. The major changes to the 1.5 million frozen meals eaten daily in New York schools were phased in over several years. In the first year there was a reduction in sugar, both at the table and in prepared food, so that sugar provided no more than 11% of calories in the diet. In the second year the use of synthetic food colourings and flavourings was stopped. After a third year had passed, improvements in academic test results took the city's average out of the bottom 40% of scores from all the states and into the top 45%.

The theory behind the changes is not that sugar and food additives are directly responsible for poor school performance, but that a reduction in 'overconsumption malnutrition' will result in better academic results. This means replacing highly processed 'empty calorie' foods with foods containing a higher ratio of nutrients to calories, so that any malnutrition present would be lowered. The increase in vitamin and mineral intake may have enabled the children to learn better and modify their behaviour, because nutrients are essential for brain biochemistry. They also responded positively to the attention being paid to them!

One study of British schoolchildren who supplemented their diets with vitamin pills has claimed an increase in IQ when measured in non-verbal tests. Subsequent tests have not substantiated the original findings; however, children with very poor nutritional status and low intake of vitamins and minerals did show general improvements in performance once they had a course of vitamin supplements, although their IQ scores did not improve significantly.

Reference Nutrient Intakes (RNI's) for vitamins and minerals

RNIs are thought to provide for most people's needs, even those with higher than average needs, so it is unlikely that anyone eating the amounts in the following tables would be deficient. However, a controversial theory suggests that the amounts need to be increased to reach optimal levels of health, aimed at preventing degenerative disease and protecting us from environmental pollution rather than just preventing symptoms of deficiency.

REFERENCE NUTRIENT INTAKES FOR VITAMINS (PER DAY)

AGE	Vitamin A (ug)	Vitamin B1 thiamin (mg)	Vitamin B2 riboflavin (mg)	Vitamin B3 niacin (mg)	Vitamin B6 pyridoxine (mg)	Vitamin B12 (ug)	Folates folic acid (ug)	Vitamin C (mg)
Males								
11-14 years	600	0.9	1.2	15	1.2	1.2	200	35
15-18 years	700	1.1	1.3	18	1.5	1.5	200	40
19-50 years	700	1.0	1.3	17	1.4	1.5	200	40
Females								
11-14 years	600	0.7	1.1	12	1.0	1.2	200	35
15-18 years	600	0.8	1.1	14	1.2	1.5	200	40
19-50 years	600	0.8	1.1	13	1.2	1.5	200	40
Pregnant	+100	+0.1	+0.3	~	~	~	+100	+10
Lactating 0-4 months	+350	+0.2	+0.5	+2	~	+0.5	+60	+30
over 4 months	+350	+0.2	+0.5	+2	~	+0.5	+60	+30

~ = no increment   # last trimester only

Source: *Dietary Reference Values*, Department of Health, 1991

REFERENCE NUTRIENT INTAKES FOR MINERALS (PER DAY)

AGE	Iron (mg)	Calcium (mg)	Zinc (mg)	Magnesium (mg)	Phosphorus (mg)	Potassium (mg)	Selenium (ug)	Sodium (mg)
Males								
11-14 years	11.3	1000	9	280	775	3100	45	1600
15-18 years	11.3	1000	9.5	300	775	3500	70	1600
19-50 years	8.7	700	9.5	300	550	3500	75	1600
Females								
11-14 years	14.8	800	9	280	625	3100	45	1600
15-18 years	14.8	800	7	300	625	3500	60	1600
19-50 years	8.7	700	7	270	550	3500	60	1600
Pregnant	~	~	~	~	~	~	~	~
Lactating 0-4 months	~	+550	6.0	+50	+446	~	+15	~
over 4 months	~	+550	2.5	+50	+440	~	+15	~

~ = no increment   # last trimester only

Source: *Dietary Reference Values*, Department of Health, 1991

Food, additives and bad behaviour

Back in the 1980s, when aversion to food additives was at the height of fashionable food fads, much bad behaviour was blamed on junk food diets. In one study at a detention centre in Alabama, in the United States, juvenile offenders who were put on a wholefood diet showed a 45% reduction in antisocial behaviour. Food additives and artificial sweeteners were removed from their diet, which previously had been based on high fat, high sugar, processed and 'junk' foods. Similar trials in Los Angeles produced a 44% decrease in antisocial behaviour, and the city council banned processed foods from its juvenile institutions.

CHAPTER 4

28 day healthy eating plan

Notes on the menus

The menus match recommendations for healthy eating (see plate guide, page 46). Most of the calories come from the 'non-fattening' starchy food group (bread, potatoes, pasta, rice and other cereals). There are five or more portions of fruit and vegetables per day, plus two or three servings of dairy foods and meat and alternatives. Fats are kept to a minimum. If hungry, serve larger portions of potatoes, rice, bread, vegetables and fruit.

The menus are not written in stone. Mix and match according to the food available, but do so bearing in mind the following:

1 Variety is the spice of life – and also of a 'healthy' diet. The 28 day menus list many food choices that could be made. The wider the variety of foods eaten, the wider the intake of vitamins and minerals. However, most people have about ten or so favourite main meals which they rotate, so you are not expected to eat exactly what is listed below.

2 When planning menus try to choose from the four main food groups in the right proportion. See plate guide and tables in the previous chapter.

Quantities

The amount will depend on appetite and age. For example a 12-year-old girl will probably require only one round of sandwiches at lunch time, while an 18-year-old boy might need two plus some soup.

Lunches

Where larger quantities are required, add variety by serving two different sandwich fillings, or a round of sandwiches and a filled roll. Or, to make things simpler, if, for example, you are serving egg sandwiches, fill one round with egg and cress, one with egg and tomato and one with egg, cheese and salad. Where the menu suggests, for example, soup and sandwiches for lunch, to avoid waste offer only one of the options if this is more suitable. However, do remember that growing teenagers should have large appetites – during their growth spurts they can easily eat twice as much as adults.

Always add at least one piece of fresh fruit to the lunch suggestions below plus, where appropriate, vegetable sticks (carrot, celery, peppers, cucumber etc) or salad. Coleslaw and bean salads transport well.

An occasional (once or twice a week) bag of lower-fat crisps is fine. Cut back gradually if this is a problem. Also add a cake or buns, such as suggested in the snack chapter, but only if the sandwiches or soup or main part of the meal is being eaten.

A yogurt or fromage frais is another good addition at lunch time. Some 'dry' granola-style breakfast cereal can be provided too, with the yogurt. Or try a mini-carton of cereal and mini-carton of milk, where appropriate.

Part of the lunch may be eaten as a mid-morning or afternoon snack. If this is the case, adjust the amount given per day. For example, do not provide a mid-morning and mid-afternoon snack if the lunchbox additions will result in over-eating or wasted food.

Puddings

LUNCH no puddings are indicated on the menu, but on a daily basis serve one or two of the following: fruit, yogurt, fromage frais, muesli bar/flapjack (not every day), fruit cake, malt loaf, spiced fruited bun, fruit scone.

EVENING MEAL no puddings are included in the 28 Day Menu.

There are several reasons for this:

- larger main courses are nutritionally better than a small main course and a pudding
- the day's menu includes regular snacks to suit teenagers' eating habits. The snacks given are more nutritious than most puddings

However, if puddings are needed choose from:

fresh fruit salad (occasionally with ice-cream) · canned fruit salad · dried fruit compotes · bread and butter pudding · rice pudding with added fruit · pancakes filled with mixtures of fruit purées/yogurt/fromage frais/fresh and dried fruit · (home-made) fruit crumbles and sponges · sweet toasted sandwiches (raisin bread filled with ricotta cheese and candied peel) · apple (or other fruit) strudel (made with low-fat filo pastry) · real fruit jellies · paneforte (see recipe) · fresh fruit fools (made with reduced fat cream or Greek yogurt or custard, not double cream) · fruit brûlées (made with thick yogurt, not cream) · reduced-fat ice-cream · sorbet · fruit kebabs · fruit tarts

Shopping guides

BREAKFAST CEREALS wholewheat cereals such as Shredded Wheat and Puffed Wheat or porridge oats are naturally high in fibre and do not contain added sugar and fat, so they are good choices. However, teenagers who do not eat a well-balanced diet, and who do not eat enough fruit and vegetables, will obtain valuable vitamins and minerals from fortified breakfast cereals (ie those that have added vitamins and minerals). Of fortified cereals, those with lowest sugar levels include Weetabix (and some own-brand versions), some corn flakes, Readybrek and Nestlé Shreddies. Others to consider are some no-added-sugar (or low-sugar) mueslis and Quaker oat bran crispies (not fortified). Ring the changes with Raisin Splitz, Kellogg's Common Sense, Weight Watcher's Perfect Balance and Kellogg's Sustain. Frosted and other obviously sugary and fatty cereals aren't the best choices – 'crunchy' usually indicates high fat and/or sugar content! There's no need to add sugar to breakfast cereals.

MILK skimmed is the lowest fat choice, but most people prefer the taste of semi-skimmed. Both skimmed and semi-skimmed contain more calcium than full fat milk, but without as much harmful saturated fat.

BREAD enjoy a wide variety of breads on a daily basis. Wholemeal and other wholegrain breads are probably the best choice for everyday use, interspersed with rye, Granary, sourdough, white, mixed grain and so on.

SPREAD whether you choose low fat or a margarine or spread high in polyunsaturates or butter, use it sparingly.

FLOUR use wholemeal or unbleached white or a mixture of the two.

FRUIT JUICE choose unsweetened juice.

EGGS use organic or free-range, where possible.

MEAT use organic or free-range, where possible.

PRESERVES use small quantities. If preferred, choose no-added-sugar jams and marmalades. Or substitute freshly made thick purées of dried fruits (apricot, pear, peach, mango), stored in the fridge, for preserves.

RICE choose wholegrain brown rice for everyday use, but use other varieties too (see Day 5 for suggestions).

SALAD use as wide a selection of green leaves and other salad vegetables and other vegetables as you can lay your hands on. Include all types of lettuce and fresh herbs, watercress, other cress, rocket, lamb's lettuce, spinach leaves, chicory, radicchio, celery, tomato, cucumber, carrot, beetroot, peppers, fennel. Add sunflower and pumpkin seeds, nuts and pine kernels. As much variety as you can muster is the key.

SUGAR sugar used in baking is raw cane sugar (eg muscovado/molasses), for flavour, but white may be used.

YOGURT/FROMAGE FRAIS try to find as 'pure' a yogurt as you can for everyday use. Many contain cheap fillers such as sugar, thickeners, modified starch, gelatine and other additives such as artificial sweeteners, and are pitifully lacking in real fruit pieces – so in fact they do not taste at all pleasant. The same can be said about a lot of fromage frais. Add your own fruit to natural yogurt. COOKING FATS use vegetable oil (eg sunflower, corn, soya, groundnut) or olive oil and butter. Limit saturated fats such as hydrogenated vegetable fats (block margarine), lard, ghee and palm oil.

Organic and free-range foods are preferable, for enviromental and welfare reasons and probable nutritional benefits.

Methods

MAKING SANDWICHES there is no need to add spread to the bread, especially if you add as much salad or grated vegetables as you can to each sandwich.

HYGIENE wash and dry hands before you start. Cover cuts with plasters. Use a clean board and knife. Wash all salad items well in cold water, drain and pat dry.

FOOD SAFETY always check use-by dates on fresh produce and adhere to them, especially where younger children are concerned. For summer consider a cool bag or a sandwich box with a built-in ice-pack facility, to keep food fresh and prevent warm temperatures at which food-poisoning bacteria multiply. Lunches prepared the night before should be stored in the fridge overnight. Check that your fridge is the right temperature – no warmer than 5°C on the top shelf.

PACKING FOOD wrap cheese (and other fatty foods) in greaseproof paper, not clingfilm. Wrap sandwiches in non-pvc clingfilm to keep the bread fresh and the filling moist. Store in the fridge until needed (eg overnight). Chill drink bottles and cartons overnight before putting them in the lunchbox.

Drinks

The best choices are water, milk, drinking yogurt, and fruit and vegetable juices. Limit the amount of fizzy and other soft drinks, whether they are sweetened with sugar or artificial sweeteners. If tea or coffee are drunk, intersperse with the above drinks. Try decaffeinated drinks and herb/fruit teas.

IMPORTANT Take changes to your diet slowly. If the Day Plans are too far removed from your present diet, step back and first make changes along the lines suggested to improve the Teenage Food Diaries in chapter 1.

28 Day Healthy Eating Plan

* indicates recipe given on pages 81-87

Day 1

Breakfast	Snack	Lunch	Snack	Evening Meal	Snack
Juice/fruit Cereal with fruit and milk Toast/bread	Milk Digestive biscuit	Lean burger* Bun Salad	Peanut butter and banana sandwich*	Pasta with vegetable and meat/fish sauce	Yogurt

Day 2

Breakfast	Snack	Lunch	Snack	Evening Meal	Snack
Juice/fruit Boiled/ poached egg on toast Extra toast/bread	Yogurt drink* Fresh fruit	Lentil*/ vegetable soup Cheese and tomato sandwiches	Potato farl sprinkled with water warmed under grill and topped with lean rasher grilled bacon/ anchovy fillets	Grilled trout New potatoes 2 servings of vegetables	Breakfast cereal and milk

Day 3

Breakfast	Snack	Lunch	Snack	Evening Meal	Snack
Juice/fruit Porridge made with milk and sweetened with 1 tbsp raisins/other chopped dried fruit, or 1 tsp honey/black treacle Bread/toast	Popcorn* Fruit juice/fruit	Egg and watercress sandwiches Twiglets	Teabread/ brack or barm bread	One pot liver casserole*/ pan-fried liver Mashed potatoes 2 servings of vegetables	Breakfast cereal and milk

Day 4

Breakfast	Snack	Lunch	Snack	Evening Meal	Snack
Back rasher(s) bacon and tomatoes, grilled Toast Extra bread/toast	Milk shake Fresh fruit	Rice salad*	Krisprolls with flavoured cottage/soft cheese	Lasagne* Add generous amounts of vegetables and pulses to the sauces 2 portions of vegetables	Nuts and raisins (small bag)

Day 5

Breakfast	Snack	Lunch	Snack	Evening Meal	Snack
½ grapefruit and prunes Milk/yogurt drink Bread/toast	Cheese scone Fresh fruit	Ham, tomato and watercress sandwiches	2 or 3 grilled fish fingers	Kebabs* made with diced pork/lamb threaded with vegetables Rice/pitta bread	Trail mix (eg banana chips, coconut flakes, nuts and seeds)

Day 6

Breakfast	Snack	Lunch	Snack	Evening Meal	Snack
Juice/fruit Scrambled eggs on toast Extra bread/toast	Sultana pancake/ Welsh cake/ drop scone	Tuna sandwich made with tuna in brine (drained) mixed with soft/cottage cheese, sweetcorn kernels, chopped celery	Muesli with milk, topped with fresh fruit (eg berries such as raspberries, blueberries)	Chilli con carne/similar mince and bean stew with vegetables Rice More vegetables	Fresh fruit

Day 7

Breakfast	Snack	Lunch	Snack	Evening Meal	Snack
Juice/fruit Apple and raisin muffin(s)*	Spring roll(s)	Smoked tofu, soft cheese and alfalfa sprouted seed sandwiches	Panforte* (or from Italian shops, delicatessens)	Sausages (low fat or grilled to drain off fat) Mashed potato Onion gravy 2 green vegetables	Toast

Day 8

Breakfast	Snack	Lunch	Snack	Evening Meal	Snack
Fruit/fruit juice Dried fruit compote with vanilla yogurt Toast/bread	Malt loaf Fruit juice	Hummus, grated carrot and lettuce sandwiches	Fresh dates and chunks of celery filled with soft cheese	Roast chicken* Potatoes 2 portions of vegetables	Apple shortcake* and spiced apple

Day 9

Breakfast	Snack	Lunch	Snack	Evening Meal	Snack
Juice/fruit Poached mushrooms and poached egg on toast Extra bread/toast	Snack pack of dried fruit (eg prunes, mango, pineapple, papaya, peach, apple etc) Fruit juice	Cheese sandwiches made with walnut bread, soft cheese, grated hard cheese, chopped apple (or grapes)	1 or 2 chicken satay sticks	Mushroom risotto* served with grated Parmesan cheese Salad	Malt loaf

Day 10

Breakfast	Snack	Lunch	Snack	Evening Meal	Snack
Juice/fruit Baked beans on toast (topped with cheese/a poached egg, if liked) Extra bread/toast	Hot cross bun/similar fruited bun	Taco shells/tortilla (corn or flour) filled with refried beans or salad and grated cheese	Tomato juice Celery sticks and carrot sticks	Vegetable curry with dahl (lentils or pulses)/ meat/fish added Naan bread/rice Raita (yogurt and mint sauce)	Twiglets

Day 11

Breakfast	Snack	Lunch	Snack	Evening Meal	Snack
Juice/fruit Raisin/bran muffin(s)	Small slice of vegetable and cheese pizza	Pitta bread filled with chickpeas and salad	Toasted raisin bread	Stir-fried vegetables with small amount of lean meat (eg chicken/ pork/beef) Rice	Fruit scone

Day 12

Breakfast	Snack	Lunch	Snack	Evening Meal	Snack
Juice/fruit Toast/bread with lean ham	Fruit cake	Fish finger Potatoes Green vegetables	1 vegetable samosa (preferably oven-baked, not deep fried)	Shepherd's pie 2 portions of vegetables	Yogurt/ fromage frais

Day 13

Breakfast	Snack	Lunch	Snack	Evening Meal	Snack
Juice/fruit French toast* flavoured with cinnamon	1 or 2 felafels*	Prawn and soft cheese sandwiches with chopped pineapple/ chives	Krisproll with slivers of Edam Grapes	Haddock grilled/ poached Potatoes 2 portions of vegetables	Instant low-fat custard with chopped fruit

Day 14

Breakfast	Snack	Lunch	Snack	Evening Meal	Snack
Milk drink Hot waffle* topped with fruit purée/1-2 tsp maple syrup	Thick vegetable soup Crispbread(s)	Baked potato with beans (baked/chilli/ other) Salad	Ryebread/ pumpernickel spread with soft white cheese topped with strawberry halves	Fish cakes Potatoes 2 portions of vegetables	Pineapple yogurt shake*

Day 15

Breakfast	Snack	Lunch	Snack	Evening Meal	Snack
Juice/fruit Toasted teacake with spread	Sardines/ similar oily fish (eg mackerel, pilchard, tuna) on toast or sardine sandwich	Pasta and bean salad made with cold cooked pasta, cooked/canned beans (eg red kidney/ borlotti/pinto) and diced vegetables of choice tossed in a small amount of vinaigrette dressing	Boursin-style cheese mixed with low-fat soft cheese, on tomato halves, grilled	Quiche Baked potato Salad	Fruit

Day 16

Breakfast	Snack	Lunch	Snack	Evening Meal	Snack
Fruit juice/fruit Banana and cinnamon pancake(s)*	Walnut bread thinly spread with mild blue cheese such as Cambazola	Vegetable burgers in a bun with salad	Date slice*	Home-made pizza* with a selection of toppings to suit all tastes Salad	Rice pudding (canned/in a carton) with fresh fruit stirred in

Day 17

Breakfast	Snack	Lunch	Snack	Evening Meal	Snack
Juice/fruit Kedgeree made with rice mixed with smoked fish and hard-boiled egg or vegetarian version with toasted almond flakes and egg	Open sandwich of 1 slice of bread, traditionally rye/pumper-nickel, topped with salad and prawns/a rollmop herring	Toasted sandwich filled with grated cheese, sliced mushroom and sweetcorn kernels	Guacamole Low-fat corn chips to dip	Meatloaf 2 portions of vegetables Rice	Bread sticks (grissini)

Day 18

Breakfast	Snack	Lunch	Snack	Evening Meal	Snack
Juice/fruit Natural yogurt mixed with crunchy muesli and wheatgerm (optional)	Potato skins Tzatsiki dip	Ham (lean) salad Bread/potato	Pinwheel sandwiches thinly spread with taramasalata	Minestrone soup (meal-size portion) Crusty bread	2-3 fresh dates Walnut halves

Day 19

Breakfast	Snack	Lunch	Snack	Evening Meal	Snack
Juice Half a papaw (papaya) with lime juice squeezed over. Parma ham Crusty bread	Slice of carrot cake (plain loaf type, no frosting or 'cream' filling)	Feta salad made with chopped feta cheese, sliced tomatoes and red peppers, black olives, chopped fresh herbs in a light vinaigrette dressing	Boiled egg Toast/bread soldiers	Meatballs with spaghetti and tomato sauce	Marmite and cottage cheese on toast

Day 20

Breakfast	Snack	Lunch	Snack	Evening Meal	Snack
Juice/fruit Bagel spread with soft cheese and topped with dill-pickled herring (in cans/jars)	Toasted Sally Lunn/teacake with cinnamon-flavoured butter	Lean roast beef/lamb sandwiches filled with lots of salad and horseradish	Black olive pâté/tapenade spread on plain cheese biscuits (eg Bath Olivers/water biscuits)	Cauliflower cheese Extra vegetables Crusty bread	Grilled banana

Day 21

Breakfast	Snack	Lunch	Snack	Evening Meal	Snack
Juice/fruit Sourdough rye bread toasted and spread with a small amount of Cambozola cheese and sliced ripe plums	Corn on the cob with butter and salt	Tomato soup Cheese sandwiches	Pasta with 1 tsp pesto sauce stirred in while hot	Moussaka (traditional lamb sauce and aubergine layers, or use potatoes instead of aubergines and a vegetarian sauce)	Peanut butter and banana sandwich

Day 22

Breakfast	Snack	Lunch	Snack	Evening Meal	Snack
Juice/fruit Cheese on toast	1 or 2 oat biscuits* Fruit	Chicken drumstick (plain or spiced, eg tandoori style) Bread/potato Salad	Smoked salmon/ smoked mackerel/tuna pâté on toast	Sausage casserole* Potatoes Green vegetable	Grilled fruit salad (eg peach, apricot, banana, mango)*

Day 23

Breakfast	Snack	Lunch	Snack	Evening Meal	Snack
Mixed fruit cocktail made from any combination of the following: grapefruit or orange segments, melon balls, strawberries, cherries, mango cubes; eat as they are, or drizzle over natural yogurt Toast/bread	Thin slice of goat's cheese on toast, melted under the grill Sliced tomato	Lunchbox salad made from a bed of crispy lettuce, apple slices (tossed in lemon juice), grape halves, slivers of cheese, walnut halves Bread roll(s)	Custard tart	Gammon steaks Mashed potatoes 2 portions of vegetables	Pretzels

Day 24

Breakfast	Snack	Lunch	Snack	Evening Meal	Snack
Juice/fruit Liver and bacon kebabs Grilled tomatoes Toast/bread	Dried apricots Milk	Vegetarian Scotch egg/ nut rissole Coleslaw Bread roll(s)	Polenta slice grilled with a paring of cheese on top	Grilled salmon steaks Potatoes 2 portions of vegetables	Simnel cake

Day 25

Breakfast	Snack	Lunch	Snack	Evening Meal	Snack
Strawberry sling made by blending 100g strawberries (washed and hulled) with 1tsp lemon juice, 2tsp runny honey, 150ml buttermilk /thin natural yogurt Toast/bread	Sour cherry muffin*	Smoked mackerel and apple salad* served on a bed of mixed salad Potatoes and/or bread roll(s)	A slice of tortilla or Spanish omelette (containing potatoes, peas and other vegetables).	Ricotta and spinach tortelloni with tomato-based pasta sauce Extra Parmesan cheese Salad Bread	Bruschetta* (Italian version of toast toppings

Day 26

Breakfast	Snack	Lunch	Snack	Evening Meal	Snack
Juice/fruit Kipper grilled without added fat. Toast/bread	Milk shake made fresh, rather than using a sugar-laden dry mixture, using any combination of fresh milk, fresh fruit and, occasionally, ice-cream	Avocado and prawn (or herring/sild/ rollmop) salad Bread roll(s)	Bread sticks (grissini)	Roast lamb (lean meat only) Potatoes Ratatouille	Pancake with fresh lemon juice and 1 tsp honey

Day 27

Breakfast	Snack	Lunch	Snack	Evening Meal	Snack
Fruit juice/fruit Family breakfast pizza* (topping below)	Cheese straws	Mackerel and chive pâté made from smoked mackerel fillets, chopped chives, lemon juice and fromage frais/Greek yogurt Vegetable sticks/toast	Sweetcorn pancake*	Grilled pork chop (trimmed of visible fat) Unsweetened apple sauce (optional in view of pudding) Potatoes 2 portions of vegetables	Baked apple filled with raisins/date mixture (see date slice recipe)

Day 28

Breakfast	Snack	Lunch	Snack	Evening Meal	Snack
Fruit juice/fruit Corn bread* Yogurt	Chinese prawn toast*	Pan bagnet* (salade niçoise in crusty bread)	Leek and cheese rosti*	Sweet and sour fish* Boiled rice	Pumpkin or sunflower seeds

Recipes

APPLE AND RAISIN MUFFINS Beat together 50g plain wholemeal flour, 75g unbleached plain flour, 1tsp baking powder, 50g sunflower margarine, 4tbsp skimmed milk, 1tsp ground cinnamon, pinch of salt and 2 eggs. Stir in 2 eating apples (peeled, cored and grated) and 50g stoned raisins. Spoon into 6 paper cases or a muffin tin and bake at 200°C/400°F/Gas 6 for 25 mins or until an inserted skewer comes out clean. Cool on a rack for 10 mins before serving while still warm.

APPLE SHORTCAKES Mix 250g plain flour, salt, 2tsp baking powder and 1tbsp sugar and rub in 50g butter. Bind to a soft dough with 150ml milk mixed with 1tsp vanilla essence. Roll out thickly and cut out 9cm rounds. Place on a lightly greased baking tray and bake at 200°C/400°F/Gas 6 for 15 mins. Serve while warm, split and filled with spiced apple: peel, core and slice apples and cook gently in a saucepan with a buttered bottom, sprinkled with ground cinnamon, cloves and/or allspice. Add a little water to prevent burning.

BANANA AND CINNAMON PANCAKES Make a basic pancake batter by sifting 100g flour into a bowl with 1tsp baking powder. Make a well in centre and add 1 lightly beaten egg and 2–3tbsp skimmed milk. Using a fork, gradually work in flour, adding 150ml skimmed milk. Stir in a couple of sliced, ripe bananas that you have dusted with 1tsp ground cinnamon and 1tbsp caster sugar. Heat a small amount of vegetable oil in a non-stick pan and drop in large spoonfuls of batter. Cook pancakes until set on one side (2 mins), then carefully turn and cook for 1 min on the other side.

BRUSCHETTA Originally this was thick slices of 2-day-old crusty home-made Italian bread, toasted over a fire and rubbed with garlic, olive oil and sea salt while still hot, then topped with salami/ham/cheese/

vegetables. Until the 1950s bruschetta was a typical snack or mid-day meal for many Italian children and farm workers. Use your imagination and top toasted bread with any combination you like (or consult a good recipe book such as *Bruschetta* by Ann and Franco Taruschio, Pavilion).

CHINESE PRAWN TOAST Mash 50g peeled cooked prawns with a squeeze of lemon juice and some pepper. Cut the crusts off 2 slices of wholemeal bread and toast one side of each under the grill. Spread the untoasted side with the prawns and gently press some sesame seeds on top. Place under the grill to brown the seeds and heat the prawns.

CORN BREAD Lightly beat 1 egg with 120ml milk. Sift 125g cornmeal (maize flour) and 60g plain wholemeal flour into a bowl with 1 tsp baking powder. Beat the liquid into the flours and put in a lightly oiled loaf tin. Bake in at 200°C/400°F/Gas 6 for 25 mins or until risen and golden and an inserted skewer comes out clean.

DATE SLICE Put 350g dates with grated rind of ½ lemon and 90ml water in a saucepan. Heat gently, stirring occasionally, until mixture is soft. Stir together 250g plain wholemeal flour, 100g porridge oats and 150g melted butter or margarine; sprinkle half of oat mixture into a 27x18cm shallow cake tin and press down well. Cover with dates; sprinkle remaining oat mixture over and press down firmly. Bake at 200°C/400°F/Gas 6 for 20 mins. Cool in tin and cut into slices.

FAMILY BREAKFAST PIZZA Spread base with 4tbsp passata (sieved tomatoes) and sprinkle on topping: 50g lean bacon, diced; 1 cold cooked sausage, sliced; 50g mushrooms, thinly sliced;. and a 125g pack mozzarella cheese, thinly sliced. Carefully crack an egg into centre and bake at 220°C/425°F/Gas 7 for 10–15 mins.

FELAFELS Drain a 400g can of chickpeas and put in food processor with ½ onion, 1 garlic clove, ½ red pepper, 1tsp ground coriander, 1tsp ground cumin and 2tbsp chopped parsley. Blend to a fine paste, roll into small patties and bake at 180°C / 350°F / Gas 4 for 20 mins or fry in oil for 5 mins. Drain on kitchen paper and serve hot.

FRENCH TOAST Lightly beat 1 egg and 4tbsp milk (enough for 2 people). Soak bread in mixture on both sides. Dry fry in non-stick pan or melt a little butter or heat a little oil in a pan and cook bread until browned on both sides. Drain on kitchen paper.

GRILLED FRUIT SALAD Place a selection of fruit (eg peach, apricot, banana, mango) on foil under a hot grill. Baste with lemon juice and when cooked through dust lightly with icing sugar.

KEBABS Marinate meat in a spiced yogurt sauce for Indian flavour, or sweet and sour soy sauce mixture. This also allows meat to be cooked quicker. Blanch or partially cook vegetables, if preferred (eg covered in microwave on full power for 3 mins). Thread vegetables and meat on skewers and cook under preheated grill. Vegetable choice: cherry tomatoes (no need to precook) onions/mushrooms/peppers/courgettes/ aubergines/mange-touts/broccoli or cauliflower florets/carrot shavings (take off with peeler).

LEAN BURGER Extra lean mince (eg 75g per person beef/pork/ lamb/chicken/turkey) mixed with grated onion, carrot, breadcrumbs and chopped tomato. Flavoured with mustard and/or fresh/dried herbs, seasoning, tomato purée. Form into burger shapes and grill.

LEEK AND CHEESE ROSTI (per person) Grate 1 medium potato, ½ leek and 15g flavoursome cheese (eg mature cheddar, Parmesan, Gruyère, emmenthal). Squeeze excess water from the grated potato. Mix the ingredients together. Heat a little oil in a non-stick pan and press the potato mixture into a cake shape in the pan. Cook for about 3-4 mins on each side.

LENTIL SOUP Chop 1 onion and 1 garlic clove and sauté in a little vegetable oil until soft. Chop 2 large carrots and add to pan with 50g any type of lentils (washed and picked over to remove stones). Cover with 400ml vegetable stock and simmer for 15–20 mins (split red lentils), 20–40 mins (brown or green lentils) until lentils are tender. Season to taste; purée or press through mouli/sieve for smooth soup, or leave whole.

MUSHROOM RISOTTO Soak 50g dried mushrooms (eg porcini) in water for 15 mins. Heat 15g unsalted butter in a pan and sauté 1 chopped onion and 2 sliced celery sticks. Stir in 250g risotto rice and stir over heat for 5 mins until rice is opaque. Stir in mushrooms and strained soaking liquid, plus 600ml vegetable stock and simmer for 20 mins until rice is cooked and liquid absorbed. Remove from heat and stir in 2tbsp chopped fresh parsley and 4tbsp grated Parmesan cheese. (Add vegetables for variety.)

OAT BISCUITS Mix 100g oatmeal, 50g plain wholemeal flour, 25g demerara sugar and 1tsp baking powder in a bowl. Rub in 100g margarine. Stir in 1 beaten egg and enough milk to make a stiff dough. Roll out on a floured surface and cut out about 16 biscuits. Put on a lightly oiled baking tray and bake at 190°C/375°F/Gas 5 for 12–15 mins until golden. Cool and crisp on a wire rack.

ONE POT LIVER CASSEROLE Slice 1 or 2 scrubbed potatoes, 1 small onion and 1 small apple (per person). Lightly oil a heavy-based pan and layer potato, onion and apple in it. Slice about 150g liver (per person) and lay on top. Pour over 150ml stock or passata (sieved tomatoes), put on lid and cook over low-moderate heat for 20–25 mins.

PEANUT BUTTER AND BANANA SANDWICH mash a small banana with 2 tsp peanut/other nut butter and a squeeze of lemon/lime juice. Use as sandwich filling.

PAN BAGNET Split open a roll or crusty French bread; rub with a halved garlic clove and brush with olive oil. Fill with sliced tomato, red onion, green pepper and hard-boiled egg. Add flaked tuna and/or anchovy fillets and black olives and season.

PANFORTE Use 100g each toasted and chopped hazelnuts and almonds, 225g candied fruit (orange, lemon, citron, melon), 100g candied peel, 2tsp ground cinnamon, ½tsp ground nutmeg, ½tsp ground cloves, 125g unbleached plain flour, and 125g each clear honey and brown sugar. Line base and sides of a 20cm square/round cake tin with rice paper. Mix nuts, peel and fruit with spices and flour. Warm honey and sugar together until sugar dissolves, then bind dry ingredients with honey mixture. Press into lined tin and top with another layer of rice paper. Bake at 150°C/300°F/Gas 3 for 30 mins. Remove from oven and cool in tin; when cold store in an airtight container.

PINEAPPLE YOGURT SHAKE (Serves 2) Whisk 400g pineapple chunks (previously well chilled) canned in natural juice with 50g natural yogurt and 2tsp runny honey in a food processor until smooth. Pour into glasses and drink at once.

PIZZA Pizza bases are easy to make. Sift 450g strong plain flour into a mixing bowl and stir in a pinch of salt and a sachet of dried easy-blend yeast. Pour in 300ml lukewarm water mixed with 1tbsp olive oil. Knead for 5 mins, then cover and leave either all day in fridge, or in a warm place for an hour or so. Roll out to make 4 pizza bases and add a topping. For example: spread base with passata (sieved tomatoes) or tomato purée and chopped herbs. Top with sliced vegetables (peppers/tomatoes/onions/mushrooms/courgettes) or sweetcorn kernels/grated carrot. Add some ham/sliced sausage/tuna/anchovy fillets and finish with with sliced mozzarella (pizza) cheese. Bake at 220°C/425°F/Gas 7 for 10–12 mins.

POPCORN Heat 1tbsp vegetable oil in a large pan with a well-fitting lid. When hot, but not smoking, remove from heat, add 100g popping corn, put on lid, shake well and return to medium heat. Shake pan occasionally while corn pops (you will hear it hitting inside of saucepan lid – do not remove!). After 3 or 4 mins all will go quiet. Remove pan from heat. Remove lid and allow to cool slightly before seasoning with salt/herbs/Marmite/clear honey. Stir well. Store popcorn in an airtight container.

RICE SALAD Ring the changes with different cooked rice (eg long-grain brown/wild rice/wild rice mixes/red Camargue rice/Jasmine rice, whatever takes your fancy). Add a wide variety of chopped vegetables (eg celery/carrot/peppers/cucumber/spring onion/red onion) plus sweetcorn kernels/chopped hard-boiled egg/flaked fish (eg smoked mackerel).

ROAST CHICKEN Do not add extra fat. Start roasting bird on its breast; turn it over (breast uppermost) for last half of cooking time. Roast on a trivet in a tin to allow fat to drain away. Pour off fat before making gravy (use vegetable cooking water); remove skin before serving.

SAUSAGE CASSEROLE Chop 1 onion, 1 red pepper, 1 large carrot and 2 sticks celery and sauté with 50g sliced mushrooms in a little oil in a saucepan for 5 mins. Add 8 pork or vegetarian sausages and stir well for 10 mins. Pour in 300ml passata (sieved tomatoes) or a 400g can chopped tomatoes. Continue to cook for about 25 mins, stirring occasionally.

SMOKED MACKEREL AND APPLE SALAD Skin 1 smoked mackerel fillet (per person) and flake into large pieces. Dice 1 apple and 1 celery stick. Add a handful of raisins and mix all together with some reduced-fat mayonnaise, lemon juice and seasoning.

SOUR CHERRY MUFFINS Lightly oil a muffin tin or use 8 paper cases. Sift 175g unbleached plain flour, a pinch of salt and 2tsp baking

powder into a bowl. Stir in 75g dried sour cherries and 1tbsp sugar. In a
jug lightly beat together 300ml buttermilk, 1 egg, 1tsp vanilla essence
and 50g melted butter or margarine. Fold buttermilk mixture into dry
ingredients and spoon into muffin tin or paper cases. Bake at 200°C/
400°F/Gas 6 for 20 mins.

SWEET AND SOUR FISH Add 1 sliced courgette and 50g
mangetouts/green beans to sweet and sour sauce (see below) or heat 350g
jar of sweet and sour sauce. Stir in 450g skinned and cubed coley fillets,
cover and simmer for 10 minutes.

SWEET AND SOUR SAUCE Mix together in a saucepan 150ml orange
juice, 150ml water, 4tbsp soy sauce, 2tbsp demerara sugar, 2tbsp wine
vinegar and 1tbsp tomato purée. Heat until starting to boil, then stir in
2tsp cornflour slaked in a little cold water. Return to the heat and stir
until thickened.

SWEETCORN PANCAKE For one, sift 40g plain flour into a bowl
with a pinch of salt. Add ½ beaten egg and enough milk to make a batter
the consistency of single cream. Stir in 2-3tbsp sweetcorn kernels and
1tbsp grated cheese (eg well-flavoured cheese such as Gruyère or
Parmesan). Make as for Banana and cinnamon pancakes,

WAFFLES Sift 50g each plain wholemeal and unbleached white flour
and 1tsp baking powder into a bowl. Make a well in centre and add 2
lightly beaten egg yolks and 150ml skimmed milk; stir the flour in
gradually. Fold in 50g melted sunflower or soya margarine. Whisk 2 egg
whites until they form firm peaks and fold them in gently. Heat waffle
maker and place 2tbsp mixture in the base; close the lid and cook for 2
mins. Alternatively use a non-stick frying pan brushed with minimal oil
and cook for 1 minute on each side.

Eating for sport – the basics

Eating a lot of starchy foods is important for sportspeople. During exercise lots of energy is needed. Carbohydrate (especially starchy) foods are the best source of fuel for working muscles, so they should make up the bulk of the diet.

For most serious sportspeople 60–70% of total energy should come from carbohydrates (but only around half for the rest of us). It's not possible to get all carbohydrate from starch so some sugar is needed. Choose 'healthy' sources eg cereal, museli bars, custard, rice pudding etc. Here are some tips to boost starchy food intake:

- Cut bread thicker and eat more of all varieties.
- Make rice, pasta and potatoes the main part of your meals and fill up on them. Try different shapes and colours of pasta for variety. Experiment with sweet potatoes, plantains and cassava
- Breakfast cereals make an excellent any-time snack.
- Eat lots of fruits and vegetables.
- Spread teacakes, scones, currant buns with dried fruit purée, jam or honey rather than spread.
- Add beans, lentils, pulses and vegetables to casseroles and sauces.

In long-term training programmes with at least one hour's strenuous exercise each day, a carbohydrate meal should be eaten soon after the session has finished. This replenishes the glycogen energy stores that training removes from the working muscles. Snacks might be easier to eat after training, followed by a meal later on. Food is probably better than sports drinks based on sugars such as glucose, sucrose or maltodextrins because food also contains vitamins, minerals and fibre.

Training also increases protein needs, but if enough calories are eaten your protein needs should take care of themselves. To recap, the main protein foods are meat, offal, poultry, fish, eggs, milk, cheese and yogurt; however, vegetable foods also contain protein, particularly pulses (beans, peas, lentils), nuts and seeds, soya products and soya milk. Even starchy foods such as bread, potatoes, pasta, rice and breakfast cereal contain protein. So you should not go short. Check with a dietitian or your trainer if in doubt.

Even though some sports call on fat reserves there is no need to eat a lot of fat. A low fat/high carbohydrate balance to the diet is right for both health and for sports performance. Sportspeople should not eat more than 30% of calories from fat (as we have seen, the average in Britain is just over 40%). To cut back on fat:

- choose low fat spread
- do not add fat to bread
- use skimmed or semi-skimmed milk
- use low-fat yogurt, soft cheese and fromage frais
- trim all visible fat off meat and eat poultry without skin
- eat more fish in place of meat
- remove fat from gravies and sauces
- avoid fatty snack foods

During hot and sweaty training fluid is lost through evaporation, to prevent overheating. Drinking plenty of water before and after exercising, and small amounts of water during is enough for most people. However, during heavy training special sports drinks that contain carbohydrate (sugar) and/or sodium may be advisable. These drinks help to speed up water absorption.

Some athletes weigh themselves before and after training to see how much liquid they need to take to rehydrate: weight loss in kilogrammes equals the litres of water required. Be sure to weigh without sweaty clothes!

- Drinks to take: water or a mixture of half water and half fruit juice.
- Drinks to avoid: tea, coffee and colas because they contain caffeine which has a diuretic effect, resulting in more liquid loss. For individual advice consult a state registered and accredited sports dietitian.

Eating for teenage pregnancy – the basics

A good diet in pregnancy is much the same as at any other time. Regular meals are essential, but eating for two does not mean eating twice as much. Quality is more important than quantity. That means choosing nutritious foods packed full of vitamins and minerals and low in fat and sugar.

Pregnant teenage girls are particularly vulnerable to nutrient deficiencies because the extra nutritional demands of pregnancy come on top of the teenagers' high nutritional demands to meet their own growth. And often they have been eating a poor diet before pregnancy, so the body is already poorly nourished. If morning sickness is experienced there are no 'reserves' for the growing baby and mother to draw on. Difficulties may be even greater if teenage girls are unaware that they are pregnant, or are trying to disguise it so that they are not meeting the nutrient needs of their baby or themselves. If changes are not made to improve the diet, the outcome is likely to be low-weight babies whose health may be disadvantaged.

Good foods for 200 calories

Women aged 19–50 need 1,940 calories a day. Only 200 extra calories a day are required during the last three months of pregnancy. Some good food choices include · 2 slices of wholemeal bread/toast with low-fat cheese · jacket potato with 30g of cheese · 1 slice of cheese on toast · wholemeal fruit bun or muffin with low-fat spread and small amount low-sugar jam · 2 bananas · 4 fish fingers · prawn/canned salmon and salad sandwich (no mayonnaise) · bowl of porridge with a few raisins stirred in · potato scone/farl with lean grilled baconrasher · cup of soup and slice of bread · just over 25g nuts · large oatcake · bagel with low-fat soft cheese

First things first

The first practical step, before any decisions are made, is to start taking folic acid supplements; 400 micrograms (mcg) or 0.4 milligrams (mg) each day. This will reduce the risk of spina bifida. For the first 12 weeks of pregnancy, folic acid supplements are available free on prescription. Continue to eat foods rich in folic acid such as green vegetables and fortified bread and breakfast cereal. For more information ring folic acid freephone helpline: 0800 665 544.

Food safety during pregnancy

Vitamin A is dangerous to your baby in the amounts found in supplements (even in multivitamin tablets) and liver. You will not go short if you eat orange and green fruits and vegetables rich in beta-carotene which is turned into vitamin A in the body. For examples see chart on page 54. Also avoid eating liver and vegetarian pâté, ready-to-eat salads and poultry, and ripened soft cheeses such as camembert, brie and blue-veined varieties. They may contain high levels of listeria. To avoid salmonella poisoning don't eat raw eggs or foods made with uncooked egg (home-made ice-cream, mayonnaise, mousses, cold soufflés). Make sure poultry and raw meat are cooked thoroughly, and take care when handling raw poultry and meat. Make sure ready or cook-chill meals are piping hot. To avoid toxoplasmosis do not eat raw or undercooked meat, always wash vegetables and salads thoroughly, and wash hands after contact with cats and kittens. Avoid all alcohol, especially in the early stages of pregnancy. One or two units a week later in the last part of pregnancy may be acceptable.

SEVEN STEPS TO EATING WELL DURING PREGNANCY	
STEP ONE:	EAT MORE bread, cereal, potatoes and pasta At least eight servings a day, more if you are hungry CHOOSE high-fibre breads and cereals NOT too much added fat
STEP TWO:	EAT MORE vegetables, fruit and fruit juice At least five servings a day, including fresh, frozen and canned vegetables and fruits CHOOSE those canned in juice, not syrup Regularly choose orange and green fruits and vegetables
STEP THREE:	ARE YOU EATING ENOUGH milk, cheese and yogurt? Three servings a day CHOOSE low-fat versions whenever you can
STEP FOUR:	ARE YOU EATING ENOUGH lean meat, fish, poultry and vegetarian alternatives? Two servings a day. Eat a variety of these foods. Try to include oily fish (sardines, mackerel, herring, tuna, salmon) once or twice a week CHOOSE low-fat versions whenever you can, eg not white fish fried in batter. Steam, grill or poach instead. Don't eat more than 4–6 eggs a week. Cook eggs thoroughly
STEP FIVE:	ARE YOU EATING TOO MUCH fat? Around three servings a day. Serving = 1 tsp margarine or butter, 2 tsp low-fat spread, 1 tsp cooking oil, 1 tsp mayonnaise, vinaigrette or other salad dressing CHOOSE low-fat spread or a margarine and cooking oils, high in polyunsaturates or monounsaturates
STEP SIX:	ARE YOU EATING TOO MUCH sugary and fatty food? eg crisps, chocolate, cakes, biscuits, fried food and pies. Try to limit to one or two a day. These foods may fill you up but they are poor nutritional value and will make you put on too much weight
STEP SEVEN:	DRINK ENOUGH Drink 6–8 glasses of water a day. You need it for the extra blood you are making for yourself and the baby, for amniotic fluid, and to prevent constipation. Replace some or all diuretic and stimulant drinks, such as tea, coffee and fizzy drinks, with water or diluted fruit juice, or fruit/herb teas

CHAPTER 5

The good snack guide

Teenagers need plenty of calories and nutrients to grow and snacks are often necessary. But most snacks eaten by teenagers are high in fat, sugar and salt and low in essential nutrients.

Around 60% of children eat at least one packet of crisps a day, with one fifth of children eating two packets daily and 14% three or more packets daily. Chocolates and sweets are eaten at least once a day by more than half of teenagers, and 13% eat them four or more times a day. Around 60% of teenagers drink cola or similar drinks at least once a day, and more than one fifth are drinking four or more cola drinks a day (11% of these are also taking an additional six or more teaspoons of sugar added to already sugary food). Around 40% of children have a takeaway meal or snack at least once a day, with a quarter eating chips once a day and 9% twice a day.

There are better choices to be made. For a gradual change towards tastier healthier snacks eat more nutrient-dense foods like those listed.

Five star snacks

- fruit – fresh, dried, canned
- vegetables – raw, cooked
- bread – all varieties including nut and fruit breads, muffins, toast, sandwiches
- breakfast cereal
- beans on toast
- yogurt and fromage frais
- soup
- custard

- popcorn
- pretzels
- potatoes, rice and pasta
- meat – lean meat (eg ham) and small amounts
- fish – canned fish (eg sardines, pilchards etc) on toast
- eggs – boiled or poached, with or on toast
- nuts, plain – in small amounts, they are high in 'good' fat, therefore high in calories
- seeds (as for nuts)
- scones, currant buns, teacakes and other low-fat cakes
- lower fat biscuits
- crispbreads
- fruit juice
- milk (and low-fat milkshakes)
- yogurt drinks

Plus all the 3-snacks-a-day suggestions in the 28 Day Eating Plan

Three star snacks

- domades (stuffed vine leaves filled with a savoury rice mixture)
- boreks (filo pastry parcels stuffed with meat/feta cheese/rice and nuts/pine kernels)
- spring rolls (oven baked)

No star snacks

- takeaways (see page 100)
- cream and cream-based desserts and toppings
- chocolate and chocolate bars
- chocolate-covered bars
- confectionery
- chips and fries
- cakes
- biscuits
- ice cream
- crisps and other savoury snacks
- fatty meat and meat products such as luncheon meat, pâté, meat pies, sausage rolls
- pies and pasties
- fried foods (eg samosas, onion bhajis)
- sugar – and in drinks
- packet puddings
- sweets
- soft drinks

Secrets of successful snacking

Fatty foods, such as 'no star snacks' provide lots of calories but without many or any vitamins and minerals. Which is why they are often called 'naughty but nice'. By all means continue to enjoy them, but not at the expense of a balanced diet. Because fat makes food extra palatable it is easy to eat more fat than is good for us.

When buying snack foods, ready meals and canned and packaged foods read the ingredients label to avoid foods that are full of sugar, modified starch, water and other cheap 'fillers' that lack vitamins and minerals. The higher up the list the more there is of that ingredient.

Crisp swaps

Limit the number of packets of crisps eaten if they are crowding out more nutritious foods, or if there is a weight problem. A standard 28g packet of plain or flavoured salted potato crisps contains around 130 calories (the fancy 'hand-fried' crisps contain more), compared with around 105 calories for lower or reduced fat crisps. That's a little – but not a lot – less. Make calorie savings with nuts. Compare a small 50g bag of roasted salted peanuts, at 325 calories, with lower fat (30% less fat) roasted salted peanuts at 250 calories: a saving of 75 calories. Plain unroasted peanuts contain the same calories as roasted, but a 50g packet of peanuts and raisins is only 230 calories: a saving of 95 calories.

Incidentally, the British spend £1.6 billion a year on crisps and snack foods. According to a survey of the snacks market by KP Foods, 6% of crisps are eaten as a result of boredom – which adds up to £96 million a year. That's an awful lot of pocket money... which could be better spent.

Chip swaps

A medium portion of 150g straight-cut oven chips 'costs' around 300 calories, compared with 430 calories for straight-cut chips, deep fried. Crinkly cut chips and French fries are higher in fat and calories.

Biscuit swaps

Lower fat/calorie biscuit choices are small digestive, Rich Tea, Morning Coffee, fig roll, Petit Beurre, Garibaldi and Nice. Some of these also come in fat-reduced versions.

Let them eat cake

Yes, but not any old cake. These are 'wholesome' fruit cakes, teabreads and muffins that make nutritious snacks.

FRUIT CAKE Line a 20cm cake tin with greaseproof paper. Cream together 100g butter or margarine and 20g dark brown sugar. Beat in 3 eggs, one at a time, adding a little of a the 250g plain wholemeal flour if the mixture curdles. Fold in 50g chopped nuts (eg almonds/hazelnuts/pecans/walnuts) and 150g dried fruit (eg raisins/currants/apricots/dates). Fold in the rest of the flour, sifted and the bran returned, plus 1 tsp mixed spice and a few drops of natural vanilla essence. Bake at 150°C/300°F/Gas 2 for 30 minutes, then lower the temperature to 130°C/250°F/Gas 1 and continue baking for about 1 hour or until an inserted skewer comes out clean.

DATE AND WALNUT BREAD Cream together 50g each of butter or margarine and dark brown sugar. Stir in 50g each chopped dates and walnuts. Lightly beat an egg and blend in. Fold in 100g plain wholemeal flour, sifted and the bran returned. Place in a small loaf tin and bake at 180°C/350°F/Gas 4 for 25-30 minutes.

MALT LOAF (less sticky for teeth than bought ones) Put 25g margarine, 2 tbsp molasses, 3 tbsp malt extract and 150ml milk in a saucepan and stir until melted together. Sift 200g flour and 2 tsp baking powder into a mixing bowl and stir in 100g raisins. Pour in the liquid and mix well. Spoon into a lightly oiled small loaf tin and bake at 180°C/350°F/Gas 4 for 45 minutes or until an inserted skewer comes out clean. Cool in the tin on a wire rack.

PUMPKIN BREAD Sift 500g strong bread flour (with malted grains, if liked) into a mixing bowl and stir in 1 sachet easy-blend dried yeast and a pinch of salt. Pour in 300ml warm water and 2 tbsp olive oil, and add 200g cooked mashed pumpkin (squash). Knead for 5 minutes (this is easier if started off in a food processor with a kneading hook). Leave to rise for 1 hour, then knock back and shape into a loaf or put in a large (1kg) loaf tin. Bake at 200°C/400°F/Gas 6 for 50 minutes to 1 hour, or until an inserted skewer comes out clean and the loaf falls easily from the inverted tin and sounds hollow when tapped on the base.

Let them eat breakfast cereal

A study of almost 5,000 16- and 17-year-olds showed that those who ate breakfast cereal regularly had a significantly lower fat diet and a higher intake of beneficial B vitamins. Slimmers and faddy eaters in particular could benefit from breakfast cereal snacks at any time of day or night. For best choice cereals, see the 28 Day Healthy Eating Plan page 68.

Incidentally, eating breakfast cereal as an evening snack does not allow you to save time in the morning by skipping breakfast, which one of the teenage diary participants thought!

Sugar myth

The idea that sugar is essential for energy and is a useful pick-me-up is a myth. Sugar added to low fibre foods, sugary snacks such as sweets, chocolate, biscuits and soft drinks may produce a quick rise in blood sugar levels and a short-term energy boost, but it doesn't last long, resulting in craving for more sweet snacks. Far better foods for energy are starchy (carbohydrate) foods such as wholemeal bread, buns, pasta, rice and potatoes. These foods produce a longer lasting energy (which is why marathon runners and sportsmen and women eat them) and they also provide vitamins and minerals for added vitality. The body gets all the 'sugar' it needs, in a 'healthier' form, when it digests these foods.

The more often sugar and sugary foods are eaten the greater the risk of tooth decay. The worst scenario being eating sugar both at meal times and between meals – a typical eating pattern for teenagers.

Soft drinks such as sugary, fizzy and fruit drinks (even undiluted fruit juice taken regularly between meals) are even more dangerous for teeth. The high acid and sugar content of soft drinks causes dental erosion where enamel and dentine are attacked and dissolved. This is far more difficult to treat than dental decay where where the hole can be filled. While the latest government survey of *Children's Dental Health in the UK* (1993) shows decreasing levels of dental decay (probably due to greater use of fluoride toothpastes), dental erosion is increasing. All sugary drinks, including fruit juice, are best taken as part of a meal to reduce the risk to teeth. Between meals, water or milk or very diluted fruit juice are best. Drinking with a staw reduces contact with the teeth.

The best drinks

Water is the original thirst quencher. If it's not fashionable, make it fashionable. Get a designer bottle or a sports bottle with sippy straw.

Water varieties to try:

- drink sparkling or still water, plain or flavoured (without sugar)
- dilute fruit juices (not fruit drinks – because they are full of sugar, sweetness and/or additives) with water
- try fruit teas and herb teas.

Other good drinks:

- milkshakes – made with fresh fruit whizzed or mashed in; flavour with real vanilla essence or fruit juices, fruit yoghurt;

whizz in iced lollies (home-made real fruit juice ones)

- yogurt drinks – better than many soft drinks, even though some contain too much sugar; home-made are good too
- flavoured soya milk drinks – these are better tasting than plain soya milk (choose calcium-fortified, low-sugar varieties)
- grain coffees or other alternatives made from barley and rye sold at health food shops – they have distinctive flavours and you may find one you love!
- decaffeinated coffee
- home-made lollies or ice sticks – get the bags from suppliers such as Lakeland Plastics (tel: 05394 88200).

Girls – low-calorie drinks and desserts

To cut down on sugar, for example in drinks and on breakfast cereal, consider an artificial sweetener. Diet and low-calorie drinks and desserts contain them rather than sugar. But artificial sweeteners may not help a lot with weight control. There is evidence that eating carbohydrate foods naturally suppresses the appetite and influences food choice at the next meal, so that a protein food is chosen to naturally balance the diet. However, artificial sweeteners may not influence the appetite in the same way which can lead to compensating, or over-compensating, by craving more sweet foods to supply the calories that the artificially sweetened food did not!

While artificial sweeteners might have a role in maintaining weight loss for people who have been overweight, the best option for teenagers is to prevent weight problems by limiting intake of too many fatty and sugary foods in the first instance.

Boys – beer and takeaways

High fat meals eaten at night do not seem to trigger effective appetite control mechanisms the following day to compensate, so adolescent boys who like beer and late-night takeaways beware of developing a seriously unsexy 'beer gut'.

Takeaway swaps

Takeaways contain a lot fat and calories so snacking on them frequently could just displace healthier foods and increase weight. Limit the number eaten and make the best choices (below).

CHINESE

USUAL Spare ribs in barbecue sauce (300g) 550–850 calories
SWAP Spring roll (200g) or fried egg roll (100g) 400–475 calories
saving 150–575 calories
USUAL Sweet and sour pork or beef (325) 700–1000 calories
SWAP Beef or chicken chow mein (325g) 400–500 calories
saving 200–600 calories
USUAL Deep-fried breaded king prawns (100g) 490 calories
SWAP Prawns without batter stir-fried and lightly dressed in soy sauce 270 calories
saving 220 calories

INDIAN

USUAL Chicken curry, eg chicken madras (200g) 800 calories
SWAP Chicken tikka masala or similar dry cooked meat curry (200g) 345 calories
saving 365 calories
USUAL Special fried rice (225g) 550–800 calories, or Pilau rice (225g) 400 calories
SWAP Steamed or boiled rice (225g) 250 calories
saving 150–550 calories

GREEK

USUAL Doner kebab (225g) and salad 750 calories
SWAP Shish kebab (225g) and salad 500 calories
saving 250 calories

PIZZA

USUAL Large deep-dish pizza (400g–550g) 800–1400 calories
SWAP Medium thin-crust pizza (250g) 500–650 calories
saving 150–900 calories

BURGER

USUAL Halfpounder, or two burgers in bun with cheese 750–900 calories
SWAP Plain burger in bun or Quarterpounder with relish etc 260–400 calories
saving 350–640 calories

FRIES/CHIPS

USUAL Thin cut French fries (150g) 475 calories
SWAP Thick cut chips (150g) 430 calories
saving 45 calories

FISH AND CHIPS

The best way to save on fat/calories is to eat the fish and leave the batter! Or cook the fish by a different method.
USUAL Cod in batter (150g) and chips (150g) 510 calories
SWAP Fresh cod fillet (100g) grilled with lemon juice and black pepper, served with new potatoes (75g) 390 calories
saving 120 calories

SCAMPI

USUAL Deep-fried breaded scampi (100g) served with 2 tsp tartare sauce 320 calories
SWAP Peeled scampi (no batter) grilled with lemon juice and black pepper 225 calories
saving 95 calories

CHAPTER 6

Why dieting is not a good idea for teenagers

We hear a lot about the dangers of being overweight from magazine articles, tv and radio programmes, newspapers and health education material. So, why do adults try to stop teenagers dieting?

It's true that weight problems are on the increase. Between 1980 and 1993 the number of obese men increased from 6% to 13% and women from 8% to 16%. At this rate by the year 2005 around 18% of men and 24% of women will be obese. Half the adult population is overweight.

But measuring obesity during childhood and adolescence is difficult. In the teenage years the body is growing and developing, which means you are going to put on weight. During the adolescent growth spurt the rate of growth is equivalent to that in early infancy. (See charts on facing page.) At its peak boys grow about 10cm a year to a total of 20cm between the ages of 12½ and 15½. Girls peak earlier, between 10½ and 12½, and grow by about 11cm during growth spurt. Growth continues into the teens for girls and and to the early 20s for boys.

Weight also increases, with girls gaining more fat to muscle than boys so that the adult male body is about 12% fat and the adult female body about 23% fat. As weight and height are gained so

Height Gain

cm/yr

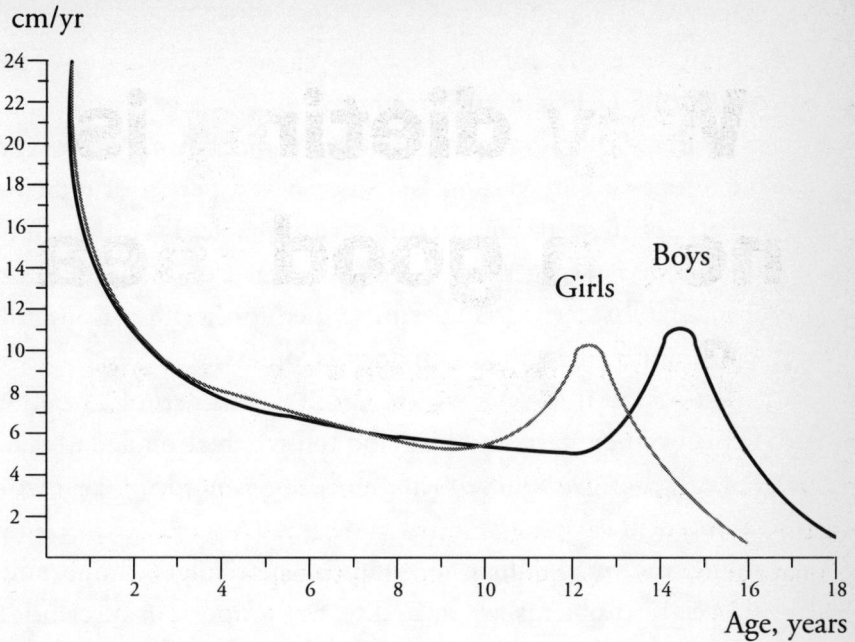

Age, years

Weight Gain

kg/yr

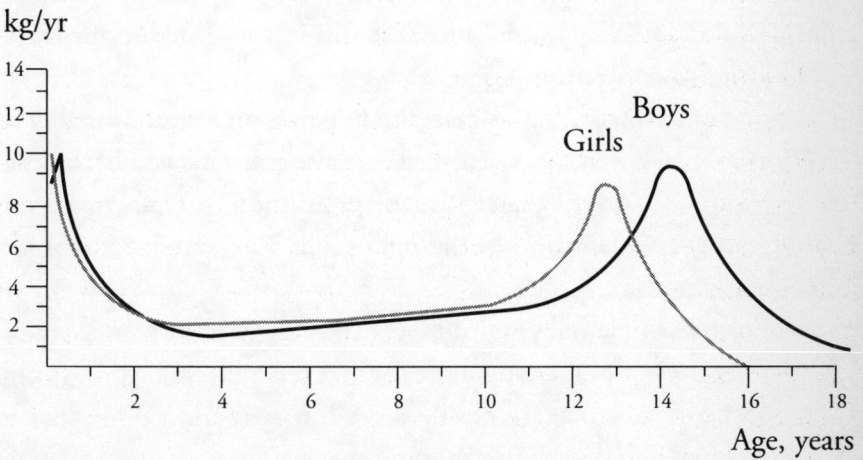

Age, years

Source: Nutrition and Teenagers, National Dairy Council Fact File 5, based on Standard from birth to maturity for height, weight, height velocity and weight velocity: British Children, Tanner et al, *Archives of Disease in Childhood* 1966; 41:454-471.

shape changes, with boys becoming broader in the shoulders and girls depositing fat around the hips, breasts and upper arms. It is normal and necessary for the body to change in this way. The greatest increase in height and weight for girls occurs between the ages of 15 and 19. So it's important not to panic! Putting on weight does not mean you are getting fat. Since it is a period of growth, wide variations in weight and height are acceptable. Even though it is suspected that teenagers who are overweight may have weight problems as adults, teenagers are still advised for health reasons not to go on slimming diets unless on doctors' orders.

The best option is to eat a well-balanced diet as part of a healthy lifestyle (ie avoid cigarette smoking and too much alcohol, and take plenty of exercise), without reducing the calories needed for growth and development.

Avoiding too many high-fat foods is particularly important because weight problems are related to the proportion of calories eaten as fat. If you eat a lot of fat you are likely to put on weight, especially if you are not very active. However, it is important not to get this message out of proportion and exclude all fats and foods that contain fat. We all need some fat – in fact it's fine for one third of calories to come from fat.

Eating a 'balanced diet' is better than going on a slimming diet if you need to lose weight. A balanced diet also prevents you becoming overweight – as every dieter knows, prevention is far better than cure. Eating a wide variety of the right foods will leave less room for 'fattening' foods.

Whatever people tell you to the contrary there is only one way of becoming overweight: eating more calories (energy) than you use up. This seems not to make sense because during the last 30 years we have gradually reduced the amount we eat, yet there are more overweight people around today. Teenagers today eat fewer calories than teenagers a generation ago; teenage girls in 1989 were eating 1.5% fewer calories than teenage girls in 1979. So why are some people heavier? The answer lies in lifestyle as much as in diet. We are simply more sedentary. We use cars and other motorised transport, and mechanised equipment and energy-saving appliances around the home, where we used to walk, cycle, run and do heavy work. And during our leisure time many of us just sit around watching tv.

Although genetic factors make some people more likely to become overweight than others, there is a lot you can do to keep your weight in check. The younger you are, the easier it is to take advantage of the two principal ways of staying in shape.

1 Increase all forms of physical activity.
2 If it's high, reduce the fat content of your diet, replacing fatty foods with starchy foods that give you lots of energy plus vitamins and minerals (bread, pasta, rice, potatoes, vegetables and fruits). Reducing the fat content of your diet helps prevent over-eating because fats tend to be less satiating (less good at satisfying hunger), and therefore are easy to over-eat.

Ten good reasons why slimming diets don't work

1 When you go on a diet your metabolic rate (the rate at which you burn calories) drops because your body adapts to the starvation of the diet by conserving energy.
2 Once you have lost weight you need to continue to eat less than you did when you weighed more, in order to maintain the weight loss.
3 If your diet did not re-train your eating habits, the weight that was lost will go back on more quickly than it was lost. This phenomenon seems to be even worse with 'yo-yo' dieting (ie spending a couple of weeks on a low-calorie diet, then stopping, then starting to diet again).
4 Slimming upsets the body's appetite and normal regulatory mechanisms for weight control. This leads to over-eating.

5 Denying yourself food, or particular foods, sets up cravings that lead to over-eating or binge eating. Restricted food intake may lead to lack of vitamins and minerals.

6 Restricting energy intake leaves dieters lethargic and lacking in energy, so they are unlikely to take exercise which helps improve body shape and tone. They will miss out on the feel-good factors that exercise gives.

7 Dieting can lead to a depression of mood and a loss of concentration.

8 Dieting leads to an obsession with thoughts of food.

9 The stress of dieting produces emotional and behaviourial problems.

10 In fact, dieting creates a whole new set of problems and is not a solution to being overweight.

To illustrate the point, in one study dieters and non-dieters were asked to take part in an ice-cream tasting. They were told that the experiment was to taste test perception of ice-cream after drinking milkshakes of particular flavours. Unknown to the participants the amount of ice-cream they ate after the milkshake was measured. The non-dieters compensated for the milk shake by eating gradually smaller amounts of the ice-creams they were given to 'taste'. However, the dieters ate more ice-cream after one or two milkshakes than when tasting after no milkshake drink.

Why does dieting have this effect?

Dieters no longer use the body's natural controls – they do not eat when hungry and when suitable food is available. The body's natural control and experience of how much food to eat are overridden. Once you stop responding to hunger cues, you are in danger of becoming a victim of psychological effects such as guilt when violating the diet. Hence, eating can easily get out of control once the dieter does start to eat. When the dieter blows the diet they simply give up, especially if the food eaten is fattening anyway.

Dieters characteristically cannot stop eating once they have started, and indeed they seem to go completely mad and overeat right before they set a date to restart a diet. Particular or forbidden foods – those that dieters think they should not eat – are more likely to cause a break-down in the diet. Under the stress of dieting people lose sight of the long term goal and are easy prey for the temptation of attractive food put in front of them. All of this leads many psychologists to the conclusion that diets are unwise, because the way dieters become obsessed with food during 'everyday dieting' is similar to the food obsessions found in anorexia nervosa and bulimia nervosa.

Ditch the bathroom scales

Although weight problems are due to having an excessive amount of body fat, it is important to realise that some body fat is essential for health. Teenage girls who might panic at the natural weight gain which is part of growing up need reassurance that this is

HEIGHT CHART
Imperial heights with approximate metric equivalents

IMPERIAL	METRIC	IMPERIAL	METRIC
4ft 10in	1.47m	5ft 9in	1.75m
4ft 11in	1.50m	5ft 10in	1.78m
5ft	1.52m	5ft 11in	1.80m
5ft 1in	1.55m	6ft	1.83m
5ft 2in	1.57m	6ft 1in	1.85m
5ft 3in	1.60m	6ft 2in	1.88m
5ft 4in	1.62m	6ft 3in	1.90m
5ft 5in	1.65m	6ft 4in	1.93m
5ft 6in	1.67m	6ft 5in	1.95m
5ft 7in	1.70m	6ft 6in	1.98m
5ft 8in	1.73m		

WEIGHT CHART
Imperial heights with approximate metric equivalents
14 imperial pounds = 1 stone
2.2 imperial pounds = 1 kilogram

IMPERIAL stone	METRIC kilos	IMPERIAL stone	METRIC kilos
5	31.81	15½	98.63
5½	35.00	16	101.81
6	38.18	16½	105.00
6½	41.36	17	198.10
7	44.54	17½	111.36
7½	47.72	18	114.54
8	43.60	18½	117.72
8½	54.09	19	120.90
9	57.27	19½	124.09
9½	60.45	20	127.37
10	63.63	20½	130.45
10½	66.81	21	133.63
11	70.00	21½	136.81
11½	73.18	22	140.00
12	76.36	22½	143.18
12½	79.54	23	146.36
13	82.72	23½	149.54
13½	85.90	24	152.72
14	89.09	24½	155.90
14½	92.27	25	159.09
15	95.45	25½	162.27

natural and normal. Many girls may have followed weight and height charts for adults and wrongly considered themselves to be overweight. Because the weights of children and adolescents fluctuate during growth, and because they have far greater needs for a high-calorie and -nutrient intake than adults, the classification of overweight and obesity in adults does not apply to them. Indeed, a broad range of weights is acceptable for people of the same height.

Body mass index figures specifically for ages 0-20 have recently been devised for use by health professionals in assessing whether young people have a weight problem. Body mass index is a far better way of assessing healthy weight than previous height and weight charts. The method is relatively height independent, so that short and tall people of similar proportions but very different weights can have similar BMIs. However it must be stressed that the method is a relatively simple index of body fatness, and it should be interpreted with caution when applied to individuals. Even though the charts overleaf are specifically for girls and boys, large but transient changes can occur during growth. These changes are normal. The charts should also not be misinterpreted for boys or girls who are very stocky and muscular and who might therefore appear to be obese on a BMI reading alone.

How to calculate BMI
Divide weight in kilogrammes by square of height in metres (m²).
For example, if weight = 25kg
and height = 1.2m,
25 ÷ (1.2 x 1.2) = a BMI of 17.4.

CATEGORY	BMI RANGE
Underweight	Less than 20
Ideal	20–25
Overweight:	25–30
Seriously overweight: you should lose weight	30–40
Definitely too fat: lose weight now	More than 40

BMI Chart (Girls)
0 – 20 years

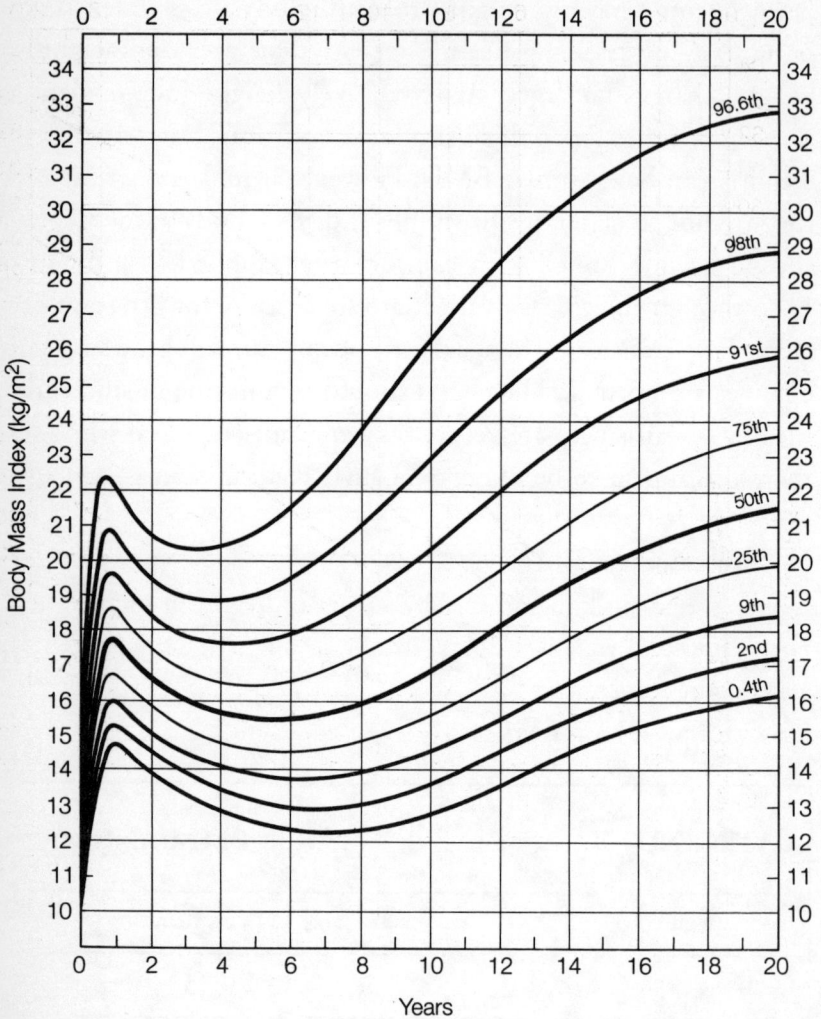

Body Mass Index (kg/m²) vs Years

Centile curves labelled: 96.6th, 98th, 91st, 75th, 50th, 25th, 9th, 2nd, 0.4th

Source: Child Growth Foundation, 1995, based on Body mass index reference curves for the UK, Cole, Freeman and Preece, *Archives of Disease in Childhood* 1995; 73:25-29. BMI and 9 centile growth assessment charts for the UK are available from Harlow Printing, Maxwell Street, South Shields, Tyne & Wear NE33 4PU.

BMI Chart (Boys)
0 – 20 years

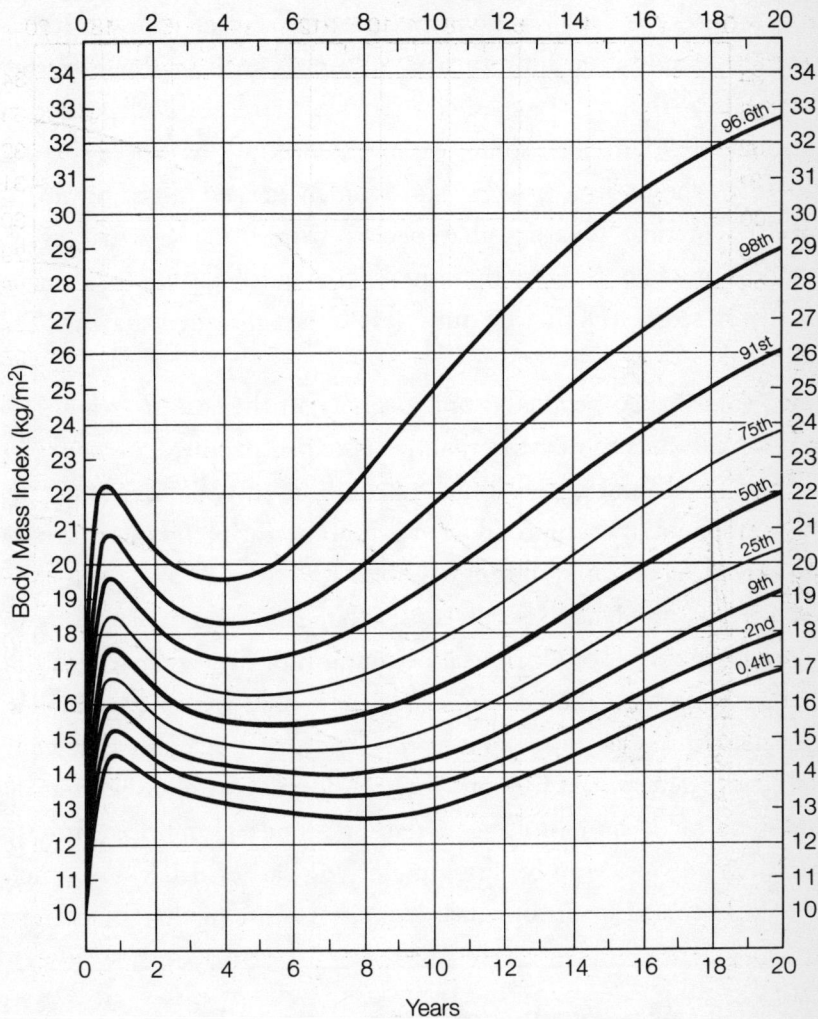

Apples and pears

We also have an in-built genetic predisposition that determines what basic shape we are: whether the essential fat on our bodies is deposited around our hips, breasts and upper arms (women) so that we are pear-shaped or whether the excess fat that is deposited is abdominal (men and some women), making us apple-shaped. However, the natural tendency for women to have slight tummies, and the cyclical bloating that occurs with the menstrual cycle, should not be confused with 'fatness'. It is quite natural for teenage girls and women to have 'tummies' (especially after having had children).

If apple-shaped people become overweight they are at greater risk of heart disease and diabetes than pear-shaped people. Excess weight caused by drinking too much alcohol is usually deposited as abdominal obesity. The good news is that increasing physical activity can specifically reduce abdominal obesity.

However, if you are basically a pear shape and you have a desire to be an apple shape, or vice versa, no amount of diet and exercise will change your basic body shape. You can only become a smaller, trimmer, firmer or more muscular version of the build that your genes have determined for you. You can do this by exercising. Eating the right foods and limiting 'fattening' foods also helps. Strictly speaking, any food can be 'fattening' if you eat (or drink) too much of it: if not used up in our daily activities some of the fat, protein

---

How many calories in your food

Fat 9 calories per gram
Alcohol 7 calories per gram
Protein 4 calories per gram
Carbohydrates (starchy foods) 3.75 calories per gram

and carbohydrate (or alcohol) will be converted into body fat. However, the most readily convertible food is fat itself. For this reason, and other health reasons, we should not overdo our intake of fat and fatty foods. But this does not mean you have to go on a slimming diet. The only reason for teenagers to avoid all fat or go on a diet is if a doctor tells them to for medical reasons.

What your best friend would tell you about dieting, if s/he knew

- Stupid comments from thoughtless people about the way we look can be very hurtful, especially to sensitive teenagers. Just because someone comments on what you are eating, or says you have put on weight, that does not mean you need to go on a diet. They are probably only trying to wind you up because they are feeling nasty, or because someone has said something unkind to them – or because they are jealous of you.
- Feeling unhappy with yourself or under pressure at home or school is not a good reason to diet. Emotional problems need airing. Stifling them by stuffing your face will only make things worse. Talk to someone, such as a school counsellor (or see Where to find help, page 177).
- Feeling dissatisfied with the way you look is natural. It happens to people of all ages, but when your body is constantly changing during the teenage years, you are bound to feel unhappy about it from time to time. Hang on in there and wait for the next change or growth spurt – like the swan, we all have to be ugly ducklings for a wee while.
- Getting grumpy about your shape and deciding to diet until you achieve the perfect shape is not going to work (see body shapes above). Regular exercise will have a lot more benefit than starving yourself, which will only make you feel ill.
- Feeling fed up about spots, bad hair days, grotty skin or whatever is your weak spot will not be solved by dieting. You

need to feed your body with nutrient-rich foods to have glossy hair, clear eyes and skin, and strong nails and teeth. Dieting deprives your body of essential and nourishing beauty foods.

• Just because your best friend, who is the same height as you, is about 3 kg (½st) lighter than you are does not mean you are overweight. We are all individuals, with our own constitutional type. Some of us will be stocky or muscular and others will have finer features and be petite. There is much beauty in diversity. Don't compare yourself to others all the time. You will feel and look even better if you concentrate on nourishing yourself from the inside out.

The dangers of crash diets

A very low-calorie diet (VLCD) that reduces calorie intake to 600 calories a day for several days or week(s) and other fad diets are not suitable for teenagers (or pregnant and breast-feeding women, children, the elderly or people with medical conditions) because they are still growing and developing. Such a diet should never be used without consulting a doctor. According to a government COMA (Committee on Medical Aspects of Food Policy) report on VLCDs, adolescents should not start a VLCD without medical supervision because of the danger of disturbing normal eating behaviour. VLCDs are typically meal replacements based on drinks and biscuits or bars; some go as low as 400 calories a day and are fortified with vitamins and minerals.

The key to looking and feeling good lies in being happy with yourself, accepting yourself the way you are, and enhancing your good points so that your natural vitality and healthy looks appeal to others. After all, the most successful actors and singers not necessarily the most conventionally 'beautiful'.

If over-eating REALLY is a problem

It is likely that one of two things are happening. Either you are consistently eating larger quantities of food than you burn up. Or, you are eating slightly more food than you burn up, which over a long period will result in weight problems. If the latter is the case, then it should be relatively simple to make small changes to the type of food you eat, rather than the amount – eat more starchy foods, fruits and vegetables to replace some sugary and fatty food. This is a far better and more successful approach than dieting.

If you want to improve your health, vitality and appearance, you could also increase the amount of physical activity you take.

If you are eating far larger quantities than you need you will have to examine your reasons for over-eating. It may be that as a family you eat larger amounts of food than you need. If this is the case the rest of your family is likely to be overweight too. Or, your family could be eating an imbalanced diet, that is, a diet made up of too many fatty foods and too little starchy foods, vegetables and fruits. If this is the case, then the whole family would benefit from making changes (see chapter 1 and the 28 day healthy eating plan).

If, however, being overweight is not linked to family eating habits, then it might be that you are over-eating because you are seeking some sort of emotional comfort from food, or just out of habit. If food is supplying an emotional need, rather than just satisfying physical hunger, then the underlying reasons need to be examined and tackled. If this is not a subject that can be dealt with at home by discussing it with parents, try talking to an appropriate teacher or student counsellor at school or college. Check out notice boards, or ask other students to suggest a counsellor with whom you might have a chat. There are several organisations that offer assistance with eating problems (Where to find help, page 177).

If it is something that can be tackled at home, then seek support in substituting lower fat foods, and limiting puddings, fried foods, takeaways and fatty or sugary snacks to occasional treats for all the family. If everyone at home is eating a good diet, the weight that you need to lose will gradually go, without any threat to your health or nutritional status. There is no need to make changes all at once. Take it one step at a time. Get used to one change before moving on.

Before dieting, try exercise

There is a much smarter solution to teenage weight problems than dieting. In a word it is 'exercise' (as you have probably guessed by now). There is a lot of scientific evidence to suggest that teenage weight problems and obesity are partly due to a general decrease in physical activity. Teenagers in general do not charge around like they did when they were 7–10 years old (although younger age groups are also exercising less). Weight problems during the teen years are more likely due to burning fewer calories – or put another way, to using up less energy – rather than eating too much. In most cases it is far better to increase the amount of physical activity than to restrict food intake.

Most teenagers will not be in any danger of overdoing it with exercise. Levels of physical activity have decreased dramatically so that children from primary school age through to the teens take very little or no vigorous physical activity at all. British children and adolescents have very sedentary lifestyles with girls' involvement in sporting activity and the amount of physical activity declining rapidly to almost nothing after the age of 14. Studies show that many people aged 55 and above, and even above 65 years, have aerobic fitness levels higher than unfit 16-24 year olds.

How to get fitter – not fatter

There are two basic ways to go about it. The first is aerobics. Do three sessions of aerobic activity per week, each session to include 20 minutes aerobic exercise. This is the best choice if you want to become fit, and it used to be thought the only way to keep in trim.

However, as most people have not taken up the aerobic challenge, advice has been modified to launch a three-year campaign called Active for Life, starting this year (1996).

This second method of getting fit is becoming more active, more often. Sweating and panting are out of fashion; doing enough activity to get warm and slightly out of breath is in. The idea is that you become more active, and that any activity is better than none. Five 30-minute sessions of moderate activity each week is the goal: take a brisk half-hour walk each day, or, if you can, walk or cycle to school, college or work. This method is the best option for those who want to become more active rather than 'fit'.

The more active you are, the easier it will become to do everyday tasks without getting tired – giving you more energy for having fun. It's as simple as that!

Method One – Aerobics

Aerobic exercise means exercising to 60-80% of your maximum heart rate for around three 20 minute sessions a week. To calculate your maximum heart rate, subtract your age in years from 220; this gives you the heart rate in beats per minute. Measure your maximum heart rate by taking your pulse at your neck or wrist during the aerobic sessions. To start with, work to only 50% of your maximum capacity.

Choose an activity you enjoy (or think you will enjoy), for

WARNING

If exercise is new to you, don't overdo it. 'Going for the burn' is dangerous. Exercise does not have to hurt to do you good. Doing any activity that raises your heart beat and leaves you slightly out of breath is all you need do. But you can also have fun! Choose an activity you can enjoy. Better still choose several and vary them.

example swimming or cycling. Women should vary these activities with others such as walking or an aerobics class, which are both weight-bearing exercises that give protection against osteoporosis. If you already exercise regularly, perfect your technique. Make sure you are doing movements fully and properly. Half a dozen properly executed exercises will do you far more good than twice as many incorrect or partially done exercises.

Warm up and cool down correctly

Start your exercise session with some stretching, gentle movement and deep breaths in and out. This avoids injury. You can either do the stretches first, and then walk briskly or use a cycle machine or treadmill for 5 minutes to warm up. Or, incorporate the stretches while marching/stepping on the spot for 5–11 minutes. After you've finished your 'workout', do not stop immediately. Keep your legs moving gently, eg a slow march or gently stepping on the spot, while repeating the stretches.

Going for it

Vary your chosen activities each week to prevent putting too much strain on the same muscles. For example, make one session jogging, one swimming and one an aerobics class or gym session. This is called cross-training, which professional athletes use to allow different muscles to work and rest on alternate days.

Home workout

You can do your aerobics at home, either to a video, or following this routine:

1 Warm-up stretches and knee-high marching for 5 minutes
2 Dancing or running on the spot for 5 minutes
3 Skipping for 6½ minutes (45 seconds skipping, 45 seconds low stepping while you recover!)
4 Stool stepping or stair climbing for 5 minutes

What's stopping you?

The main reasons women give for not exercising are:

'I'm not the sporty type' (you don't have to be)

'I'm too shy or embarrassed' (there's no need to be, try a women's-only activity)

'I need to rest and relax in my spare time' (you will feel much more relaxed after exercise)

'I haven't got the energy' (fitter people have more energy)

'I'm too fat' (even if you are, which you probably are not, only exercise can alter the shape you are and improve the way you look in your clothes)

So what's stopping you now?

---

5 Repeat steps 2 to 5

6 Cool down stretches while keeping those legs moving.

NB If at any time you feel pain, discomfort or are too breathless, DO NOT STOP, but walk around gently until you feel able to continue.

Method Two – More Active More Often

- Try to fit a 30-minute walk in before and/or after school, college or work by getting off the bus or tube a stop earlier.
- Climb the stairs instead of using the lift or escalator.
- Leave your desk for a 5-minute walk a few times during the day – even this little bit of exercise is estimated to reduce your body fat by just under 1kg (2lb) annually!
- Try a lunchtime walk (or maybe a swim).
- What about an active evening class such as salsa dancing or badminton, or aqua-robics at your local pool?
- The busier and more active you are, the more calories you burn and the fitter you will become.

Swimming is a great exercise for women because it can be continued into pregnancy. For those not used to exercise, swimming is also easier on the heart which does not have to pump against gravity. The water also provides body support. However, for it to be effective you need to be able to swim for half an hour.

Start off with a 15-minute swim. Make up the time with 15 minutes of pool exercises or a brisk walk to the pool, or do some exercises when you get home. At the pool swim two 25-metre lengths, alternating two strokes if possible. Rest for a minute and repeat three times. Gradually increase the number of lengths each time you visit the pool until you are able to swim for 30 minutes.

Pool exercises

1 Water-jogging: run on the spot, bringing your knees as high as you can. Start with 20 steps per leg and build it up.
2 Water-jumps: stand in the shallow end, crouch down by bending your knees, touch the bottom of the pool and then jump out of the water as high as possible. Do this 10 times to start and build up the number.

Power walking This can be done for free and needs nothing more than a reasonable pair of aerobic/running/cross-trainer shoes:

1 Walk briskly for 5 minutes.
2 Jog for 1 minute, then walk for 1 minute. Repeat 10 times.
3 Walk for 15 minutes (adding short jogs, if you like).
4 Cool down stretches.

There are many benefits to walking. It strengthens the heart, muscles and bones, improves circulation and inspires creative thinking. Successful walkers cruise comfortably at 5.6km (3.5 miles) per hour (a 17-minute mile).

Shaping up – how exercise beats dieting

1 Body mass index in girls increases most between the ages of 15 and 19, making this a critical time for weight gain.
2 Teenagers are often concerned about weight gain, yet they are also very inactive.
3 Regular physical activity prevents weight problems, encourages weight loss (if needed) and improves appearance.
4 Exercise helps prevent heart disease, stroke, high blood pressure, diabetes, osteoporosis and some types of cancer.
5 Exercise is mind-bendingly good – psycho-social effects of exercise/sport include reduction of stress and depression, increase in self-esteem, elevation of mood and increased feelings of relaxation. Experience the feel good factor yourself.
6 Dieting interferes with growth and natural eating habits
7 The best thing to do at this critical time in your life is to increase physical activity.
8 Eat more starchy foods and more fruits and vegetables.
9 Eat less fatty and sugary 'junk' foods

If dieting goes too far

Many teenage girls surveyed about their eating habits have a fear of being overweight. They perceive themselves to be far

---

Don't be beaten by the boys

It is estimated that one third of men and two thirds of women would find it difficult to sustain walking at a reasonable pace (about 4.8km/3 miles an hour) up a 1 in 20 slope. They would soon be out of breath and have to slow down or rest. However, only 4% of 16- to 24-year-old men fall into this unfit category, while a staggering (literally!) 34% of women in this age group do.

heavier and 'fatter' than they actually are. In response to their dissatisfaction with their body size or shape they become highly 'restrained eaters' who frequently diet. This is a time when they should be growing and are supposed to be getting heavier not lighter. It is not surprising that the number of cases of anorexia nervosa has increased in the last 30 years, when the popular image of successful women in magazines and on tv is equated with thiness. Being inside an adolescent body that is growing in all directions (hips, breasts, bottoms) in the face of such messages from the media might make most adolescent girls wish they could step into Alice's Wonderland, reach for a bottle labelled 'drink me' and shrink to the requisite size. After all, many adults wish they had straighter backs, whiter teeth, shapelier legs, smaller noses, a bit more height, and so on.

Pressure from peer groups to be slim is given as one of the main reasons for dieting. Comments from boys and friends that girls are fat or have an unattractive body shape tend to provoke periods of dieting or slimming. This is hardly surprising when faced with the realisation that as women they will be judged on how they look. As a result they feel wary of any food that might make them overweight, and therefore unhappy and unwanted. Yet at the same time they are also preparing for roles in which they will provide food for themselves and probably for others. There is the prospect of leaving home, and there may even be a choice between having a career or becoming a home-maker. Some will feel under pressure to live up to the lifestyles portrayed in some women's magazines, in which readers are encouraged to 'have it all'.

Growing independence from parents, teachers and others may make teenagers hostile to any intervention in their slimming practices. While believing they are asserting their independence by controlling what they eat through dieting, they are also giving in to peer or social pressure to conform to a particular appearance. Building their confidence so that they are not susceptible to pressures to diet is a challenge for family and friends.

Nobody knows how to prevent eating disorders. There is no hard evidence than any one thing works. There is currently a study in progress in Norway to see if putting preventive measures into schools works. A trial in Australia suggests that even if students (and staff) know more about eating disorders, they do not occur any less frequently.

One of the dangers of diets, especially among teenagers, is that depriving the body sets up strong cravings which can lead to binge eating and other eating disorders such as anorexia nervosa and bulimia nervosa, and these need effective psychotherapy to overcome.

Symptoms of eating disorders

These are similar to the medical effects of starvation: poor concentration, an obsession with calories and food, lack of confidence, low self-esteem and denial that there is a problem.

ANOREXIA NERVOSA, which literally means loss of appetite for nervous reasons, is the relentless pursuit of thinness through self-starvation and a fear of becoming fat, it typically affects adolescent girls who are high achievers and who come from families where academic and social achievements are encouraged and valued but is found elsewhere, too. In westernised societies throughout the world it affects 1-2% of teenagers.

For anorexia nervosa to be diagnosed, a doctor checks for all the following symptoms. This is an essential guide for parents who need to act if these signs are present:

- body weight maintained at least 15% below expected (either lost or never achieved)
- self-induced weight loss by avoiding 'fattening foods' and one or more of the following: self-induced vomiting/purging; excessive exercise; use of appetite suppressants and/or diuretics
- pathological body-image distortion with a dread of fatness and

a self-imposed low weight threshold
- widespread endocrine disorders - that only a doctor will be able to diagnose
- delayed puberty (in prepubertal cases) with arrested growth so that in girls breasts to not develop and periods do not start. Parents can be assured that with recovery puberty is often completely normal, although periods start late.

There may be associated problems such as severe constipation and abdominal pain, dizzy spells and swelling of the stomach, loss of friends, emotional and irritable behaviour, difficulty sleeping, feeling cold, alopecia (loss of hair on the head), laguna growth of downy hair all over the body.

For BULIMIA NERVOSA to be diagnosed, a doctor checks for all the following symptoms:
- persistent preoccupation with eating and an irresistible craving for food so that the person binges (has episodes of overeating large amounts of food in a short time)
- attempts to counteract the 'fattening' effects of food by one or more of the following: self-induced vomiting, purgative abuse alternating with periods of starvation; use of drugs such as appetite suppressants, thyroid preparations or diuretics. Diabetics with bulimia sometimes neglect insulin treatment.
- a morbid dread of fatness. The person sets a weight threshold well below what would be considered normal. There may be an earlier episode of anorexia nervosa to varying degrees.

Family and friends may notice secretive behaviour in people with bulimia nervosa who often disappear to the lavatory after meals. Other problems associated with bulimia include menstrual disturbance, sore throat and erosion of tooth enamel caused by vomiting, dehyration and poor skin condition, lethargy, emotional and behaviour mood swings.

With both of these eating disorders the manipulation of food is an expression of psychological and emotional problems. Sufferers think they are solving problems by controlling eating. In fact, they are:
- concentrating all energies on food and eating, or not eating, to avoid other issues, or apparently insoluble problems, in their lives
- exerting control over their body, and life, when they feel other people are controlling them
- reacting to unresolved stress and problems that may go back years

It is only when they become physically ill and the eating disorder becomes the dominant problem that they begin to realise they are in difficulty.

Where to get help

The earlier anorexia nervosa is recognised and treated, the better the long term prognosis. The recovery period can be long and slow because weight gain takes time alongside psychotherapy. The family play an important part in the process, especially in the cases of younger sufferers. However, what works for one person may not be effective for another. Early recognition of bulimia nervosa is also preferable, however treatment is usually short-term with very good results.

A good starting point for seeking help is the family doctor, because in order to gain access to existing services the condition has to be diagnosed. This might be difficult if the sufferer is reluctant to admit the problem to the doctor, or if the doctor has little training or understanding of eating disorders. A few GP practices have expertise in dealing with eating disorders, but most will refer someone with anorexia nervosa or bulimia nervosa to specialist help, usually at an out-patients department of a hospital with psychiatric services, or another mental health agency. Some hospitals have specific eating disorder units or clinics.

Referring a teenager with anorexia nervosa to a specialist service with a long waiting list is dangerous because eating disorders can become severe in teenagers more quickly than in adults. Ideally adolescents should be assessed and treated by a multi-disciplinary team which is part of local child and adolescent mental health services that offer therapy involving the family. Treatment for anorexia nervosa should include some of the following elements: counselling, psychotherapy, cognitive behaviour therapy, group therapy, family therapy, day hospital programmes, in-patient treatment, dietetic advice, and support for carers. If these services are not available locally, referrals should be sought through the NHS to either NHS or private specialist centres. Most cases of bulimia nervosa are dealt with by out-patients psychotherapy or counselling services, usually on a 10-15 week programme.

What is treatment like?

A senior dietitian working at the Maudsley Hospital, which has a nationally recognised eating disorders unit, describes the treatment there:

'The first choice of treatment is family therapy, which works best for under 16s and a lot of under 18s as well. The whole family is assessed by a psychiatrist and then the psychiatrist and/or other therapist(s) treats the family. If it is not a success, or the family rejects the offer of therapy, or sessions break down, other approaches are tried.

'When a teenager with anorexia nervosa first sees the dietitian she will be asked what she thinks has happened to her weight, how long she has had weight problems, when she first became concerned about her weight, and whether she has any concerns about her condition now. The patient will be asked what eating was like as a young child as far back as she can remember, and what she did to manipulate her weight and restrict her eating and her concerns about it. Many teenagers are worried that they are doing themselves some permanent damage. The dietitian will explain what damage might be done, depending on each patient's condition, and explain the concerns about their condition.

'The next step is to work out what they can do initially to stop any further weight loss and improve the amount and quality of what is being eaten. They will then tackle together what rate of weight increase the patient could cope with and how best she could use the help offered. An eating plan would be constructed to bring about gradual weight increase using the foods the patient feels most able to eat. If, for example, the dietitian has major concerns about low calcium intake and risks of (or established) osteoporosis, then foods containing calcium would be suggested for that reason. Similarly, anorexics are often lacking iron and zinc, and it may be necessary to suggest foods containing these. During normal growth spurts of adolescence larger amounts of protein are needed.

'The foods most people with anorexia have most fear of are fat and sugar. They are usually OK with most fruits and vegetables (although some have scurvy because they do not eat any or enough of these). Starchy foods such as jacket potatoes, wholemeal bread and bran flakes are usually acceptable, as are cottage cheese, skimmed milk, beans and pulses and vegetarian foods.

'Twenty years ago anorexics would not eat starchy (carbohydrate) foods, although they would eat a lot of cheese, because the pervading slimming/health message of the time was that starchy foods were "fattening". This has subsequently been disproved, but it is interesting that anorexics, both then and now, take the general health message for the population as a whole and apply it to themselves in the extreme. Today anorexics tend to take the general healthy eating message to "limit your intake of fat and sugar" to unhealthy extremes.

'Some cases of anorexia are a temporary period of weight loss and very low weight, which occurs during the teenage years and is overcome by the help of the anorexic's family and therapy during a year or so of treatment. In other cases the girls will already have had a long history of eating disorders from childhood. Sometimes it can happen for the first time in older women, but often women in their

30s and 40s who attend out-patient clinics for treatment have also had episodes in their teens.

'If out-patient treatment is not a success, or if an anorexic relapses (one or a dozen times) she can often be admitted to hospital in a state of collapse because anorexia has made her physically ill. Some cases are seen for the first time by health professionals when they reach this state and are hospitalised. But if anorexia – very low body weight – is continued it will inevitably lead to hospitalisation eventually, because the body cannot keep well for a long period on a very low weight.

'At the Maudsley there is a 16-bed unit where the girls live together rather like at a boarding school. After medical assessment they are normally started on three meals a day, plus three snacks. If they are too frail to eat they will be started on fluids, but if they are able to eat (and most are) they will start on small, soft-textured, low-fibre low-fat meals that are not a challenge to their compromised guts. It is felt to be important to start them on "real" food from the beginning, even though some eating disorder units use intravenous (tube) feeding methods. Using these methods is thought to be invasive (especially for patients whose eating disorders stem from physical or sexual abuse), unhelpful and an unnecessary delay in getting the patient to deal with eating real food.

'After a few days a wider range of foods and more calories are introduced. By two weeks the girls will be eating 3,000 calories a day. There is a choice of foods from the beginning – the only thing the girls do not control is the amount of food eaten. There will be girls at all stages of treatment on the unit at one time and they are able to support each other.

'The teenage girls are discharged when they have reached a healthy weight, but if older women with maybe a 20-year history of anorexia are known not to be able to tolerate a normal healthy weight, they will be discharged when they are thought to be at a safe weight. All patients of the unit continue to attend out-patients for a year. Some will move into a local hostel that works with the unit if they are not able to go home. They can stay at the hospital for six months.

'Although there are probably ten times as many binge eaters (bulimia nervosa and compulsive eaters) as anorexics, the condition is more common among older women than teenagers. The best known therapy for binge eating is cognitive behaviour therapy. Binge eaters typically have no experience of normal eating. They may have eaten chaotically from a young age and do not really recognise normal eating patterns in others. They typically restrict themselves all day and then binge all evening. Or they may restrict themselves for days or a week and then binge for several days. The only patterns of eating they know are dieting and bingeing. They may have observed their parents eating three meals a day and even eaten the three meals a day with them, but then they would eat four more meals a day on their own. Somehow the normal learning process for eating has become derailed.

'Most teenagers tend to go through a process of experimentation with eating and meal patterns, to learn for themselves what suits them. They come out of it as adults with their own way of eating. Some people successfully eat two meals a day, some six – adjusted to their own nutritional and energy needs. Binge eaters do not seem to learn through trial and error. Very early on they learn to restrict and to binge. That is the pattern they know, and they are terrified to try anything else because it seems too risky. Even though their current pattern of binge eating is frightening, at least they know what to expect. It is familiar and therefore not as risky as trying to construct a pattern of eating that means frequent doses of food.

'Normally a dietitian would suggest they adopt a pattern of eating a small amount every two or three hours. They can then tolerate the gaps between the meals, and gradually build a pattern of eating four or five times a day.'

How parents can help prevent eating disorders

1. Don't panic if teenagers start to diet. For most is it a brief and benign pastime; even though it does nothing for their general health and vitality

2. Use any dieting as an opportunity to raise awareness of, and interest in, a healthy balanced diet (chapter 3) that will, over time, result in weight loss - only if it is needed

3. At the same time consider your own attitude to food, diet and other people. These attitudes may need changing if you encourage your children to admire or aim for slimness, or equate slimness with health, or have little respect for people who are not very slim.

4. Try to build teenagers' self-confidence and self-esteem. Encourage them to take a more realistic view of themselves and their body image. Ask if they really admire supermodels who compromise their health and starve themselves for money, and who will be discarded the minute they put on a pound or two.

5. Try to quash the myth that thinness will bring happiness. Happiness is more likely to come from within, from a person who feels good about themselves and makes the most of themselves as they are.

6. A sense of inner pride and self worth does not emanate from people with a constant desire to be 'made over' and whose only sense of worth is related to being slim or thin.

7. If you are worried about the possibility of eating disorders look out for tell-tale signs (diagnostic list pages 123-125). Seek professional help as soon as possible.

CHAPTER 7

How to be a healthy vegetarian

There are nearly three million vegetarians in Britain today (4.5% of the population), with teenage girls leading the statistics. There are twice as many vegetarian women as men.

Among the 16- to 24-year-old age group more than 13% of women claim to be vegetarian. This is three times the national average and three times the number who were vegetarian in 1984. Nearly one quarter of 16 to 24 year olds avoids red meat – more than twice the national average. A further four million Britons are no longer eating red meat, although they may still eat poultry, game or fish; others are cutting down on meat consumption in general. It is predicted that by the turn of the century there could be five million vegetarians and ten million non (red) meat eaters in Britain. These predictions were made before the current BSE in beef crisis, which might turn more teenagers against meat.

The risk from BSE

The unusual deaths of 10 teenagers among 20 people aged under 42, from a new strain of CDJ (Creutzfeldt-Jakob Disease), have increased fears about BSE, or bovine spongiform encephalopathy, better known as mad cow disease.

Fears centre on the possibility that the disease might be transmitted to humans who would suffer it in the form of CJD. No-one can say for certain whether eating beef and beef products contaminated with the agent that causes BSE will cause CJD in humans. However it is thought that the deaths are linked to exposure to BSE before a ban on bovine offal was introduced in 1989.

One theory about the cause of the BSE epidemic is that lower temperatures introduced in the 1980s for rendering animal offal for animal feedstuffs no longer destroyed the agent that caused scrapie (another encephalopathy) in sheep. The agent then passed to cows and cattle (which are herbivores) where it caused BSE, either in its original, or a new form. Scrapie has been present in the national sheep flock in Britain for at least 250 years without evidence of causing human health problems. BSE became a notifiable disease in 1988 after which all affected cattle were ordered to be slaughtered and incinerated. In addition, in 1989, specified bovine offals (brain, spinal cord, tonsil, intestine, thymus, spleen) were ordered to be removed from cattle over six months of age at the slaughterhouse or abattoir, dyed and destroyed. Recent enquiries suggest these controls often lapsed and that infected food may have entered the human and animal food chains. The Ministry of Agriculture says that old cattle food containing infected animal material was still being used for some time after the initial ban on its use came into effect. As BSE may have an incubation period of up to 20 years some cases may also be the result of feed eaten before the ban. The Ministry also blames more recent cases on infected foodstuffs 'leaking' into cattlefood.

In December 1995, in a move to tighten up BSE controls, the government banned the use of bovine vertebral column in the manufacture of MRM (mechanically recovered meat) as 'a precautionary measure to remove the risk of spinal cord tissue entering the human food chain', and to protect us from what they then called a 'remote theoretical risk of BSE'. Although spinal columns should have been removed and destroyed since 1989, checks by vets at slaughterhouses and abattoirs revealed that small amounts of spinal cord were being left in some carcasses used for the manufacture of MRM. Other procedures were not being carried out correctly.

In 1996 government advisers recommended that carcases from cattle aged over 30 months should be deboned in specially licensed and supervised plants and that trimmings be kept out of the food chain, and that the use of meat and bonemeal from any mammals be banned from feed for any farm animals – to prevent BSE spreading to pigs or chicken. So far there is no evidence that BSE is transmitted via the germ cells (semen/egg), but studies continue.

- BSE has never been found in milk samples tested for it.
- If the infective agent for BSE was found in red meat or other meat products, domestic cooking would not destroy it. Temperatures high enough to destroy the agent would make the meat inedible. (Examples of beef products are meat pies and sausages made with mechanically recovered meat, meat stocks and extracts and foods that contain them such as gravy granules and soups. Beef products such as gelatine are widely used to thicken yogurts and other dairy desserts, confectionery, jellies and many other items – even lipsticks.)
- Despite concerns government advice is that beef remains 'safe' and that if human infection with BSE occurs, children and groups such as pregnant women and others with compromised immune systems are not at any increased susceptiblity to infection. The Consumers Association and other consumer groups advise people not to eat British beef.

Foods to replace meat

Strictly speaking, vegetarians 'eat no fish, flesh or fowl'. Most vegetarians eat eggs and dairy produce. Vegans eat no animal produce at all. Giving up meat in itself does not automatically make a diet 'healthier'. On the other hand there is no reason why a well-balanced vegetarian diet should not supply all the needs for adolescent growth.

Meat and meat alternatives are the main source of protein in the normal diet. Protein in animal foods is made up of amino acids (protein building blocks). In meat, fish, dairy foods and eggs, the nine essential amino acids that cannot be made in the body are found in the right proportion. To get the right proportion in a vegetarian diet, a combination of two of the three plant protein food groups listed below needs to be eaten. The three groups of vegetable protein foods are:

- pulses (beans including soya beans, peas, lentils)
- nuts and seeds
- grains (rice, bread, pasta and other wheat products, rye, barley, oats)

Vegans in particular need to combine vegetable proteins. Dairy foods enhance the available protein in vegetable foods, so vegetarians who eat milk, yogurt, cheese and eggs will obtain 'complete' protein very easily.

If this all sounds rather technical, be reassured: vegetarian protein combinations come in familiar everyday foods such as beans on toast, bread and hummus, peanut butter sandwiches, dahl (lentil curries) or bean curries with rice or Indian breads, Mexican tacos and refried beans, and pasta and bean salads.

Vegetarian protein foods are high in fibre (meat, fish, cheese and eggs lack fibre) and many, especially nuts, beans, grains, seeds and soya foods, are also low in saturated fats. Other vegetarian protein foods include tofu (soya milk curd), tempeh (made from fermented soya beans), textured vegetable protein (TVP made from soya bean flour) and Quorn (a mycoprotein/fungi). With the exception of tempeh, most are available from supermarkets and health food shops. Quorn has no flavour of its own but absorbs flavours from sauces and other foods with which it is cooked. It is available as mince and chunks, and is also sold in ready-meals and pies.

With so many vegetable protein foods to choose from, it is easy to avoid the pitfall of relying too much on any one food, for example cheese or eggs. New vegetarians can tend to over-eat these, which should be avoided because they are (like meat) high in saturated fats. A well-balanced vegetarian diet can offer clear health benefits.

A teenage vegetarian in the family

When a teenager in the family or household changes their diet, for whatever reason, it inevitably has consequences for the person who buys and prepares the food – usually Mum. The rest of the family or household will carry on eating their meat and two veg, but the 'household manager' will have to change shopping and preparation habits. New types of food must be bought, and they may not always be available where the shopping is usually done. There will also be implications for the budget because vegetarians cannot just leave out the meat, or eat a chunk of cheese instead of meat, at each meal – alternative protein foods must be found (see page 134). This will inevitably mean extra work initially until a new pattern emerges to accommodate the member of the family who has decided to eat differently.

However, with many foods (eg pasta, stir-fries, grills, risottos, soups, pizzas) one basic meal can be prepared with meat or meat alternative added to the appropriate portion(s) at the appropriate time in preparation. For the change to go smoothly, all members of the family will have to adapt and make compromises, and be patient!

Health benefits of a vegetarian diet

Heart disease and cancer are still the main causes of premature death in Britain, and studies show vegetarians are less likely to get either. A good vegetarian diet is protective against heart disease because it is lower in fat and higher in antioxidants and fibre. Too much fat, and saturated fat in particular, leads to a high blood cholesterol level which increases the risk of heart attack.

Vegetarians also have lower blood pressure, which further reduces the risk of heart disease, stroke and kidney problems. Why, is unclear – it may be to do with eating less fat, or less salt, or having a better overall nutrient (vitamin and mineral) intake rather than simply because they don't eat meat. Vegetarians are less likely to be cigarette smokers, are more likely to be active and they may be less stressed, or have better ways of dealing with stress!

Vegetarian protection against the one third of cancers that are diet-related (including lung, breast and colo-rectal) may come from the fibre in cereals, and the fibre and antioxidant nutrients in fruit and vegetables – when eaten as part of a low-fat (especially saturated fat) diet. Vegetarians are also less likely to need slimming diets because they are typically leaner than meat-eaters.

Parents – ignore detractors and don't worry

Parental worries are natural when a child becomes vegetarian, especially if there is no experience in the family of catering for vegetarians. Advertisements such as one run by the Meat and Livestock Commission only serve to create unnecessary anxieties – as the Advertising Standards Authority recognised when it upheld complaints against the MLC. In the national press advertisement in question, part of a newspaper article headline: 'Your children need meat, parents told as anaemia spreads'. The article said: 'Vegetarian parents could be to blame for a growing number of anaemic children, it was suggested yesterday. A government survey of 1700 youngsters showed that a lack of red meat resulted in a shortage of iron in one in 12 of under-fives and one in eight of those aged one and half to two and a half...'

As objectors to the advertisement pointed out, millions of vegetarians live long and healthy lives, and a well-balanced vegetarian diet contains all the necessary vitamins and minerals. The objectors also said the government survey did not link red meat to the amount of iron in the body.

The evidence had shown neither that children required meat to be healthy nor that balanced vegetarian diets could be detrimental to their health, said the Advertising Standards Authority.

Some common questions about vegetarian diets

Q What is a healthy vegetarian diet?
A In essence it is the same as a healthy non-vegetarian diet. The proportions of food on the plate should be the same (see chapter 3). The only difference should be the replacement of meat, poultry and fish with vegetarian alternatives (see also protein question).

Q Will vegetarian girls become anaemic?
A Teenage vegetarian girls are more at risk than non-vegetarian teenagers of becoming anaemic through low iron intake (and sometimes low folic acid and vitamin B12). Iron-rich vegetarian foods include green leafy vegetables, pulses, tofu, eggs, dried fruit, wholemeal bread and fortified breakfast cereals. However, iron found in plant foods is less easily absorbed by the body than iron found in meat. Food or drink rich in vitamin C (citrus fruit/juices, other fruit and vegetables) with the meal will improve uptake.

Good sources of zinc (which is also better absorbed when taken with vitamin C rich food and drinks and eggs or dairy foods) include pulses, brown rice, and wholemeal and rye bread. Zinc is also found in cheese, eggs, carrots and peanuts. Eat all of them regularly.

Q Will vegetarian girls get osteoporosis later in life?

A Osteoporosis is a disease in which bones lose their mass and fracture easily. Prevention begins young (see page 55). One survey of vegetarian women between 50 and 89 showed bone loss of 18% compared with 35% among non-vegetarians. Other surveys showed no difference. To prevent osteoporosis, vegetarians and non-vegetarians alike need a good calcium intake, adequate exercise and avoidance of cigarette smoking – throughout life.

Good sources of calcium (in addition to milk, yogurt, fromage frais, cheese and eggs) are wholegrain cereals, muesli, oatmeal, pulses, nuts and seeds, dark green vegetables and dried fruit. Hard water, and some minerals waters, are also good sources of calcium. White bread is also fortified with calcium, so alternate with wholemeal.

There are many reasons why people become vegetarian. For example:

- concern about animal welfare
- health (a vegetarian diet can be lower in fat, especially saturated fat, and has other health benefits)
- fear about 'mad cow disease' and similar scares
- environmental issues
- religious and cultural issues
- dislike of meat (taste and texture)
- ethical issues such as fairer sharing of the world's food (and water) resources: fodder crops that could feed humans directly, especially in Third World countries, have to be grown to feed animals that then 'wastefully' convert them into protein. Besides which, countries that cannot or do not feed their own children and adults raise cattle and other 'luxury' crops for export to affluent countries that want cheap food

Q Why should s/he want to go vegetarian? Don't they like my cooking?

A Food is such a personal thing that other members of the household can feel rejected or threatened if one member decides to become a vegetarian. Don't take somebody else's decision personally. And do not put undue pressure on an adolescent to give up, or treat their decision as a 'five minute wonder'. Accept and support, as long as they also give and take, and help with food preparation and shopping, as appropriate.

Q Do vegetarians need to take vitamin supplements?

A A balanced vegetarian diet will supply all the nutrients needed. In fact, studies have shown that adult vegetarians have an adequate intake of nutrients, often higher than the national average. However, vitamins B12 and D are found mainly in animal foods. Vegetarians eating dairy foods seem to get enough B12. Vegans who do not eat any animal produce might need B12 supplements in addition to foods fortified with B12, eg yeast extract, some vegetable stocks, vegetable burgers, soya milk and breakfast cereal. Margarine – but not all low- and reduced-fat spread – is fortified with vitamin D. (See also page 57)

Q Will vegetarians be less brainy or be more at risk of heart disease because they do not eat fish oils?

A The special properties of fish oils help reduce the risk of heart attacks and are essential for the brain and eyes. For these reasons, non-vegetarians are recommended to eat fish twice a week, because habitual consumption reduces health risks. Fish oils contain high levels of a type of fatty acid called EPA (eicosapentanoic acid), a long chain omega-3 fatty acid. EPA, which is in turn converted in the body to DPA (docosahexanoic acid), is vital for brain and retinal function, and foetal and baby development. However, vegetarians need not go short of EPA because the essential fatty acid alpha-linolenic acid (from soya and rapeseed oils, pulses, walnuts, broccoli and green leafy vegetables) is converted in the body to EPA. EPA makes the blood less likely to clot and cause thrombosis (heart attacks). The second type of essential fatty acid is linoleic acid (omega-6 fatty acid) from sunflower oil, vegetables, fruits, nuts and cereals, which is well supplied in a good vegetarian diet.

Q Will I suffer flatulence if I eat all vegetarian foods?

A Flatulence often accompanies an increase in fibre. Switching to a good vegetarian diet means eating more pulses (beans, peas, chickpeas, lentils), wholemeal bread, pasta, brown rice and other high-fibre foods. Some people are more susceptible to wind than others, but usually the problem subsides as the naturally occurring bacteria in the gut adjust to the changes. Some people find eating more live yogurt speeds up the body's adjustment.

Q Will a vegetarian diet cost more?

A Following a vegetarian diet need not be more expensive. Many vegetarians say it is a lot cheaper as they eat more pasta, rice, beans, pulses, bread and vegetables, which are among the cheaper foods. Seasonal fruit is inexpensive, especially when it is used as a 'loss leader' by supermarkets to attract customers. Frozen vegetables, which are as beneficial as fresh, are often cheaper, eg peas and sweetcorn. Dairy foods and vegetarian protein foods, such as Quorn, soya proteins and tofu, are cheaper than lean, humanely farmed meats.

Not only does vegetarian eating cost less for individual families, it also helps the earth's resources go further, because it is cheaper and more environmentally friendly to produce vegetable crops than meat in current farming practices.

Q How can I avoid animal food additives?

A If you wish to avoid all animal ingredients you will have to become a very careful shopper; buy a reference book such as *E for Additives*

(M. Hanssen, Thorsons) and read labels.

See list of common food ingredients derived from animals Appendix, page 181.

Other foods to watch out for when shopping

BURGERS and SAUSAGES need not be made from meat. There are many frozen and chilled burgers and other 'grills' available fresh (chilled) and frozen from health food shops and supermarkets.

CHEESE (such as cheddar and other hard cheese) that is made using vegetarian rennet will be labelled as such. Vegetarian agents for clotting milk are plant or fungi enzymes or lactic acid and bacteria. Standard rennet is made from rennin, an enzyme taken from the stomach of slaughtered calves. Soft cheese such as cottage, curd, ricotta and skimmed milk cheese are made using bacteria or lactic acid.

CRISPS Not all meat-flavoured crisps are made from meat extracts. Check with manufacturers – some chicken ones, for example, are made using vegetable-based flavourings.

EGGS Look for eggs from organic or free-range systems rather than farm fresh or any of the synonyms for eggs produced from battery/intensive systems.

GRAVY MIXES that are not based on meat stock or meat extract are available from health food shops. You can also use vegetable stock (cubes) and bouillon (cubes).

MARGARINE, SPREAD or LOW-FAT SPREAD Look out for brands made from vegetable oils that are low in, or free from, trans fats and animal ingredients, and high in polyunsaturates.

MINCEMEAT (mince pies, Christmas pudding) are traditionally made with beef suet. There are several brands suitable for vegetarians made using vegetable fats.

PÂTÉ Vegetable pâtés are available from health food shops and some supermarkets.

READY-MEALS Fresh (chilled) or frozen should be labelled if suitable for vegetarians. Try to choose lower-fat ones.

SOYA MILK choose calcium fortified, sugar-free varieties. Some contain honey and sugar. If you haven't used soya milk before, follow these tips for storing: • do not dilute until the moment of use; store the remainder undiluted • transfer from can, once opened, to a non-metallic container and store covered in the fridge • once opened it will keep for up to 5 days in the fridge (unless packaging states otherwise).

WORCESTERSHIRE SAUCE This traditionally contains anchovies, but there are some vegetarian versions available from health food shops.

YEAST EXTRACTS, such as Marmite and Vegemite (the Australian version), are suitable for vegetarians (unlike Oxo and Bovril).

YOGURT The lowest fat varieties are low fat (0.5 – 2% fat) and very low fat (less than 0.5%). Check the labels of low-fat and diet yogurts for gelatine and other additives that are used to sweeten and thicken, to make them appear 'creamy'.

For up-to-date shopping details contact the Vegetarian Society or the Vegan Society (Where to find help page 181).

Genetic modification

Foods made from genetically modified ingredients are now on sale. For example, some supermarkets sell tomato purée made from genetically modified tomatoes. Many groups, including vegetarians, have concerns about genetic modification of foods and animals especially in the light of BSE problems that are a result of man interfering with nature by feeding herbivores contaminated animal protein. In the case of tomato purée the gene responsible for the enzyme that softens tomatoes has been literally turned round to switch off the softening process. The fruit is said to be able to ripen more fully on the vine to develop flavour and colour while remaining firmer for transportation and less watery for processing. This cuts processors' costs and saves water. Benefits claimed for consumers are lower price and better flavour. The government has been criticised for not making clear labelling compulsory, but so far products are clearly labelled. So if you have doubts about genetically modified foods, you need not buy.

The vegetarian meal planner

The plan contains lots of suggestions to show the variety of choice available. And, of course, if you eat a wide variety of different foods you increase your intake of vitamins and minerals. Hungry teenagers may need snacks too. For snack ideas see 28 day healthy eating plan page 66 and Good snack guide page 93.

Day 1

Breakfast	Lunch	Dinner
Fruit juice	Minestrone soup	Vegetarian burger
Shredded Wheat	Wholemeal roll(s)	Large mixed salad
Wholemeal toast	Fresh fruit	Jacket potato
		Fruit brûlée

Day 2

Breakfast	Lunch	Dinner
Fruit juice	Slice of wholemeal	Nut croquette or
Scrambled egg on	vegetable and cheese	nut roast
wholemeal toast	pizza	Carrots
More toast, low fat	Green salad	Broccoli
spread and preserve	Yogurt	Mashed potato
		Vegetarian gravy
		Fruit salad

Day 3

Breakfast	Lunch	Dinner
Muesli Stewed dried fruit Yogurt	Baked potato, Beans and/or grated cheese Fruit	Vegetable curry Dahl Brown rice Sorbet or frozen yogurt

Day 4

Breakfast	Lunch	Dinner
Poached mushrooms on wholemeal toast Milkshake	Hummus with crudite (raw vegetable sticks) crispbread or bread Fruit	Pasta with vegetable sauce Grated cheese Low fat rice pudding and dried fruit

Day 5

Breakfast	Lunch	Dinner
Grapefruit Wholemeal toast, low fat spread and preserves	Wholemeal pitta bread filled with mixed salad and chickpeas Yogurt	Paella or risotto or pilau with mixed vegetables and nuts

Day 6

Breakfast	Lunch	Dinner
Fruit juice Wholemeal hot cross bun or fruit scone Low fat spread	Toasted sandwich filled with grated cheese and tomato Watercress and celery sticks Flapjack or similar bake	Spanish omelette filled with potatoes peas and other vegetables of choice Fruit fool

Day 7

Breakfast	Lunch	Dinner
Fruit juice Porridge made with skimmed or semi-skimmed milk Stir in raisins or other fruit of choice	Baked beans on toast with cheese on top, if liked Fruit	Baked potato Vegetarian quiche/flan Mixed salad Apple crumble and custard made with skimmed milk

Day 8

Breakfast	Lunch	Dinner
Fruit juice Weetabix Wholemeal muffin Low fat spread	Carrot and nut salad Wholemeal roll(s) Yogurt	Cauliflower cheese Large mixed salad Jacket potato Fruit salad

Day 9

Breakfast	Lunch	Dinner
Fruit juice Boiled egg Wholemeal soldiers with low fat spread and Marmite	Rice salad, with sweetcorn peas and peppers Wholemeal scone	Buckwheat and vegetables

Day 10

Breakfast	Lunch	Dinner
Muesli Stewed dried fruit Yogurt	Pasta salad with canned kidney beans and broad beans, tossed in vinaigrette dressing Fruit fool	Vegetable burger or bake Ratatouille Crispy French bread Grapes and an individual mini cheese

Day 11

Breakfast	Lunch	Dinner
Fruit juice Poached egg(s) on wholemeal toast	Vegetable samosa(s) with rice or naan bread Yogurt	Pasta with vegetable sauce Grated cheese Baked custard

Day 12

Breakfast	Lunch	Dinner
Grapefruit Wholemeal toast low fat spread and preserves	Mexican taco shells filled with mixed salad and little grated cheese Fruit	Risotto with mixed vegetables and nuts

Day 13

Breakfast	Lunch	Dinner
Fruit juice Croissant without spread or preserve	Vegetarian pasty Fruit	Stir fry vegetables with tofu and sweet and sour sauce Fruit fool

Day 14

Breakfast	Lunch	Dinner
Fruit juice Sultana pancake with yogurt	Egg sandwiches with watercress or other green salad Fruit	Stuffed peppers (or other vegetables) Rice Pancakes with fruit pureé filling

CHAPTER 8

Beauty foods, stress beaters, 'healthy' drinking

If you are not yet convinced that diet and exercise will give you a better body, better looks and energy to enjoy yourself, then read on...

We all care about the way we look and the way others perceive us. Teenage girls in particular are aware of the importance of first impressions. They think if people – and especially boys – are to like them, they have to look attractive, which usually means not being overweight. Boys, on the other hand, want to be fit and muscular, although some are more relaxed about appearance. They are aware that while they base judgements about girls mainly on appearance, girls judge them more by personality.

While girls may imagine they are overweight when they are not, boys do not so readily admit to being overweight. They see extra pounds as either puppy fat, or part of their masculinity, or just the way they are. Girls, however, tend to have a far more self-critical approach to body and self image, often imagining themselves to be far less attractive than they are.

Boost your confidence

Do not under-value yourself and your achievements, whether they are academic or related to work or the home. You might think that your achievements, personality and even self-respect are invisible to others, especially when compared with the importance placed by men, boys and society at large on physical appearance. But first impressions, and how slim or attractive you are, should not be the most important factors in your life.

If you think that no-one is going to know, on first meeting you, that your have done well at school or passed your driving test first time, or have other achievements, whereas they are going to notice if you are a few pounds overweight, then think again. Anyone who judges you solely on appearance is not making a sound judgement. If they cannot be bothered to ask you about yourself, then do not bother about them. You are far more likely to make a lasting impression if you are self-confident and at ease with yourself. Other people will be far more relaxed in your company – and want to be with you – if you make the most of yourself, and your interests are more than skin deep.

Of course you want to look your best. It is perfectly natural, so long as it is not part of an obsession with body shape and weight. There are far more interesting and vital things to do during the teenage years.

It is far more important that you build your confidence, and try to be more self-reliant and not exist simply for the praise and recognition of others. When you feel good about yourself you will not want to diet, and you will learn to lose guilt feelings associated with food or obsessions about food and dieting.

This is not to say that it is 'fine to be fat' and that the health risks associated with being obese are an invention. There are definite health risks in being obese which are associated with poor food choices.

Enough said. Now it is time for a light-hearted quiz to check out your attitudes!

Teenage diet and lifestyle quiz

Few of us have totally predictable lifestyles, so answer the questions below working on an average day or week. Don't be tempted to give the reply that you think is 'correct'. Answer honestly (it pays in the long run!)

1. Good morning! It's breakfast time:
a) I'd rather spend a few more minutes in bed, so I skip breakfast.
b) I just have a coffee and maybe some crisps or chocolate on the way to work/school.
c) Grapefruit and toast, usually wholemeal, or sometimes cereal.
d) I meet my friend for a pain au chocolate at the station, or I take a cappuccino and a Danish into the office.

2. Mid-morning coffee time:
a) I'm starving, so I have a Mars bar from the vending machine or a few biscuits with coffee/cola.
b) If I haven't had a cola already, I have one now, or another coffee with my cigarette.
c) I don't often drink tea or coffee. I prefer mineral water, milk or fruit juice.
d) If I've had a bad morning, or there's a lot to do, I tend to eat more, so I might have a pastry or a couple more biscuits than I should.

3. Lunchtime:
a) I'm vegetarian so the choice is often limited. I usually have a white cheese roll or soup.
b) I go to the wine bar/out of school for lunch because there's no hassle for smokers. I usually make do with peanuts or crisps, or a burger and chips.

c) I make a packed lunch of wholemeal sandwiches, or quiche or salad. Other days I have ready-made salads or sandwiches and a yogurt drink or a fruit juice.

d) For lunch I'll have a snack such as pork pie and coleslaw, or a sausage roll, or French bread and pâté or cheese. I always have a pudding, even if it's just a custard tart or fudge cake.

4 It's evening and time for your main meal of the day:

a) If I'm going out there's not much time for cooking, so I'll have some pasta and a tub of ready-made sauce. I like fried rice with vegetables, too.

b) If I'm really hungry I'll pick up a takeaway on the way home. Otherwise we have a ready-meal: it could be Indian, Chinese or Italian.

c) Plain grilled chicken or salmon with boiled potatoes and vegetables are quickest in the week.

d) Pie and chips, sausages and mash, or spaghetti bolognese are our regular dinners. Then we'll have some ice-cream or an individual trifle or chocolate mousse. I like a hot chocolate drink and biscuits before bed.

5 Which of the following statements is closest to your exercise pattern?

a) I use public transport to cut down on environmental pollution. I might go for a walk in the park at weekends, but I don't like organised sport or go to a gym.

b) I play squash occasionally (to make up for smoking!).

c) I aim for three aerobics sessions a week, but I usually only do two, although I do go swimming once a week.

d) I always take the lift, and I arrange to meet friends at cinemas or cafés near a tube or bus. I get too puffed out and uncomfortable to walk far. In the evening I rarely leave my favourite tv armchair.

How did you do?

Few of us fit into exact pigeonholes. If your answers were, for example, mostly a) then this is your 'type'.

a) As a vegetarian you have a potentially healthy diet, but at the moment it is not varied enough. Without three meals a day it is difficult to eat enough of the vitamins and minerals needed to help you look and feel good. You should eat breakfast on a regular basis. Fruit juice, followed by fortified breakfast cereal with semi-skimmed (or no-sugar soya) milk would be good. Breakfast would give you more energy and make it easier to give up the mid-morning chocolates. Swap white bread for wholemeal at lunchtime and elsewhere, and vary the sandwich fillings to include more salad, raw vegetables (eg grated carrot), nut butters, hummus and other vegetarian fillings. In particular, you need to make one meal a day a good vegetarian protein meal. Organised games and sport at school may have put you off exercise, but it is time to grow up about this and find an activity that you enjoy. There are lots to choose from. See also chapters 5 and 7.

b) Your first goal is to give up smoking. As you are already missing meals you probably think that means putting on weight, but it need not (see page 169). At the same time try to start eating regular meals, if necessary with two hourly snacks to get you over the nicotine craving. See chapter 5 for suggestions. Until you have kicked the habit, you will probably want to continue with the stimulant fizzy drinks, but in the long term you should swap these for caffeine- and sugar-free versions because too many can play havoc with your blood sugar levels, resulting in cravings for chocolate, biscuits and so on. Regular meals will help avoid blood sugar swings, and associated mood swings and cravings. Your choice of meals is rather high in fat. If you have to rely on ready-meals, serve them with extra vegetables, rice or potatoes and choose the lower-fat versions. Well done for playing squash. Your long-term goal should be to play regularly – you will find that fixing more regular matches will help with giving up smoking. Remember to warm up and cool down properly. To avoid the sudden demands that a game like squash puts on your heart, look for a 'gentler' exercise until your fitness is established. See page 116-121.

c) OK, so you are doing everything right and annoying all your friends with your healthy and well-toned body. Keep it up!

d) It sounds as though your emotional needs are being met by food. Your goal has to be to find another 'comfort' factor in your life. Regular exercise might be part of the answer, as it will give you the highs and relaxation you currently get from food – without piling on the calories. Try to have breakfast before you leave in the morning. If you have to eat out for breakfast, choose a wholemeal sandwich or toast instead of Danishes and pain au chocolate, which should be occasional treats. Lower-fat/calorie foods for lunch include sandwiches, salads, baked potatoes, pasta or rice dishes. Your current lunchtime choices added to your evening meal choices are the equivalent of two high-fat main meals a day. Try to cut out at least one pudding a day; replace it with fruit or yogurt. Swap the bedtime drink for a lower calorie version – and eventually give it up. At the same time as changing your diet, you need to introduce some gentle exercise on a regular basis. Swimming would be a good choice; ask about 'ladies only' or 'learner' sessions at your local pool, if you are embarrassed about exercising.

Top ten beauty foods

Foods for clear skin and eyes, shiny hair and strong nails are:

1 Oily fish such as herring/salmon/sardines/trout/mackerel
2 Orange fruits and vegetables, eg oranges/apricots/peaches/ carrots/squash

3 Dark green leafy vegetables – these are packed full of vitamins and minerals
4 Milk – lower fat is best
5 Oats – in porridge and muesli
6 Yogurt – low-fat and low in sugar, if possible
7 Wholemeal bread, and wholemeal pasta/brown rice/potatoes
8 Fortified breakfast cereals that are no- or low-sugar and not fatty
9 Walnuts and other nuts and seeds in small amounts
10 Very lean red meat, including liver (unless you are pregnant)

Top beauty drink

There is no contest because there is only one – water. Drink at least a litre a day, for a clear complexion, clear eyes and overall fitness.

Eating to avoid spots

If you have spots or acne, you are not alone – only three out of ten teenagers escape unscathed. Acne varies from mild in some people to painful and severe in others. Treatments will vary according to how your skin responds.

Acne during adolescence occurs when the sebaceous glands over-produce a greasy fluid called sebum, in response to rising hormone levels. The sebaceous glands are found all over the skin, except the palms and soles, but are most numerous on the face. The pores through which sebum normally escapes become blocked, allowing bacteria to grow in the sebum, and the result is blackheads. Acne can be brought on or worsened by some medicinal drugs and moist tropical working conditions. In girls acne can worsen around the time of the period because of changes in hormone levels.

While doctors will tell you that diet does not affect acne and spots, sufferers will say it does. Chocolate in particular is said by some people to make their acne worse. If this is the case, try to avoid it for a while, or limit your intake. Even if chocolate does not cause spots, eating it leaves less room in your diet for foods that contain the nutrients needed for clear, healthy skin.

Exercise, fresh air and a good cleansing routine (for chaps of either sex!) will also help prevent spots. However, if they do occur, squeezing spots is not a good idea as it will lead to inflammation and scars. Blackhead removers are not recommended. A blackhead will come away when it is ready. Skin should be washed with normal soaps or light (non-oily) cleansers. Antiseptic face washes that kill bacteria may help. The most popular treatment is benzoyl peroxide which reduces sebum excretion, loosens blackheads and kills bacteria. Sunlight improves the condition of most acne sufferers' skin, but be careful not to get burned by the sun. Protect the skin with sunscreens that contain both UVA and UVB protectors. Sun protection factors SPF are marked on most products – the higher the number, the greater the protection.

As you progress through the teens hormones become more settled and major problems with spots lessen.

Foods to feed your skin

Throughout your teens, concentrate on building good skin from the inside. Skin needs feeding from the inside because it is being constantly shed, in a 21 to 30 day cycle. Collagen and elastin fibres keep skin supple. They are made from protein, so you need to eat enough protein, but this is not something to be concerned about. If you eat enough calories, your diet will almost certainly provide you with enough protein. In fact, most Western diets provide more than we need.

In addition, vitamins A, C and E, the antioxidant minerals copper and zinc (see good food sources of antioxidant nutrients, page 53-54), iron (protein foods), calcium (dairy foods) and B vitamins (starchy foods) are needed for healthy skin, eyes, teeth, hair and nails – all are obtained from a balanced diet.

Other tactics for great skin

SLEEP A good night's sleep (7–8 hours) makes your skin look clearer and fresher and keeps away dark circles under the eyes.
EXERCISE Glowing skin follows aerobic exercise sessions because they get the circulation going to nourish the skin.
HEALTHY DIET A well-balanced diet will feed your skin as well as the rest of your body.

Foods for bad skin

- Too many cakes, biscuits, chocolate and other confectionery
- sugar and sugary foods
- fried and fatty foods
- smoked foods
- caffeine in coffee and cola especially at the expense of more nutritious foods
- spicy food
- cigarettes and alcohol

Good looking snacks

If you are hooked on chocolate bars, crisps or other fatty and sugary foods, don't expect to give them up overnight. Cut down gradually to one a day. Then try one every other day, substituting an alternative from the list below. As you gradually change your diet (in the steps outlined above) you will find cravings for unsuitable snacks gradually disappear. Try these healthy snacks:

- fresh fruit
- no-need-to soak dried fruit
- oatcakes
- toast with low-fat spread and Marmite/cottage cheese
- crisp rolls
- fortified breakfast cereal with semi-skimmed milk
- fruit yogurt
- vegetable sticks (celery/carrots)

Foods to protect your teeth

The increase in fruit juice consumption may have boosted vitamin C intake among teenagers, who (like toddlers) seem to have an in-built antipathy to vegetables more so than fruit, but it has caused concern for teeth. Along with sugar, sugary foods and other carbohydrates, fruit juice is seen as a potential cause of dental decay.

The problem with sugar is that it feeds bacteria that live in dental plaque. The bacteria produce acid that attacks the tooth, causing caries (holes) in the teeth that need filling.

Stickiness makes matters worse, so toffees and other sugary foods that stick to your teeth are more likely to cause dental caries. Late-night sweets and bedtime biscuits are particularly bad as the flow of saliva reduces during sleep. Saliva has a role as a natural tooth cleanser; without it, sugars can ferment all night and bacteria can really get to work on your teeth. Starchy foods such as bread are also broken down in the mouth into simple sugars which can be used by plaque bacteria, but not to the same extent as sugar and sugary food.

The more frequently sugary foods and drinks are taken, the greater the risk of dental decay. Acid foods such as colas, fruit drinks and, to a lesser extent, fruit juice should also be of limited frequency. This is a problem, because they are popular among teenagers and are taken throughout the day. Using a straw reduces contact with the teeth.

Unfortunately, from the dentist's (and dairy farmer's) point of view, milk has become a less popular drink among teenagers, especially girls. In 1982 milk was the main drink among teenagers, accounting

---

Tooth-friendly snacks

Safer snacks for teeth are cheese, nuts, milk and milk products.
Less safe snacks for teeth are sweets, sugar, dried fruit, biscuits, cereal foods.

for 40% of drinks consumed by 11- to 16-year-olds; by 1993 it had fallen to 16%. The decline of milk drinking among teenagers comes at a time of growing evidence that milk and cheese may be protective against tooth decay, even in the presence of sugar. These foods seem to neutralise acids in the mouth, produced by bacteria fermenting sugars, and stop them attacking tooth enamel. The consistency of cheese, which sticks around the teeth and mouth, encourages a high concentration of minerals, especially calcium, in saliva, which may allow some damage to the tooth surface to be repaired.

Replacing the 'empty' calories in nutrient-deficient fizzy drinks and sugary drinks with nutritionally well-balanced milk, flavoured milk and yogurt drinks could give teenagers a lot to smile about in the long run.

What fate worse than false teeth?

Before they get their second teeth, more than half the children in the UK have dental decay. Adolescents continue to be at risk of tooth decay because they eat sugary foods frequently throughout the day, as the teenage food diaries for this book show. The more often you eat sugar and sugary foods the greater the risk of tooth decay. The worst scenario is to eat sugar both at mealtimes and between meals – a typical eating pattern for teenagers

Soft drinks such as sugary fizzy and fruit drinks (even undiluted fruit juice taken regularly between meals) are even more dangerous for teeth. The high acid and sugar content of soft drinks causes dental erosion where the enamel and dentine are attacked and dissolved. This is far more difficult to treat than dental decay where the hole can be filled. While the latest government survey of Children's Dental Health in the UK (1993) showed decreases in levels of dental decay (probably due to greater use of fluoride toothpastes), dental erosion was increasing. All sugary drinks, including fruit juice, are best taken as part of a meal to reduce the risk to teeth. Between meals, water or milk or very diluted fruit juice are best.

Too tired to party

Tiredness and poor academic performance in some teenagers are linked to anaemia. Lots of teenagers lounge about looking washed out. For some it is an attitude. Sadly, for others, particularly teenage girls, it is a sign of anaemia which leaves them tired all the time and as breathlessness as old ladies after exertion. Anaemia impairs intellectual performance and therefore learning and school achievement.

Low iron intake – a problem with many adolescent girls in the UK (see also chapter 2) – is the main reason for nutritional anaemia (although low folic acid and low vitamin B12 may also be involved). One study of London schoolchildren aged 12–14 found low iron and low vitamin C intake. Anaemia was three time more common in girls than boys, and a quarter of the vegetarian girls and 23% of girls who had tried to lose weight in the last year were anaemic.

What is anaemia?

Anaemia results from too little haemoglobin in the blood. Iron is part of haemoglobin, which is the pigment in red blood cells that takes oxygen to all parts of the body. If you are short of iron, your red blood cells contain less haemoglobin so your body has to work harder to supply you with enough oxygen. This leaves you feeling weak, tired and short of breath. Teenagers have a high requirement for iron, needing it for growth and to make the larger volume of blood required as the body grows. Some substances, such as phytates in raw bran and tannins in tea, bind with iron, thus preventing it being absorbed into the bloodstream. Despite this, teenagers (and adults) should not take a lot of iron supplements because too much iron can be harmful. Treat iron tablets as medicines and always stick to the recommended dose.

Is stress making you eat the wrong foods?

You don't have to be a particular age to suffer stress. Neither do you have to be a person with a high-powered job. In fact, people who wield the power are usually not under stress because they are in control of everyone and everything.

On the other hand, most people who feel stressed do so because they do not enjoy what they are doing, or they feel powerless to control their situation or environment.

Teenagers are prone to stresses because they are in a transition period from childhood to adulthood. There is a natural tension between wanting to choose your own things and live your own life, and the restrictions imposed by home, school, college and the law.

The stresses about limits, rules and regulations imposed by parents (and schools) can erupt into family rows about going out. Parents naturally want to know exactly where teenagers are going and with whom and what time they will be home, and teenagers want to just go and come back when they like.

Teenage stress quiz

Find out how much stress you are under.

1. Image – are you:
   a) unhappy with the way you look?
   b) worried that you are not fashionable enough?
   c) constantly having 'bad hair' days and spots?
   d) plagued by criticism about the way you look?

2. School/work – are you:
   a) confident that you will achieve what you need/want?
   b) about to take important exams/move, or lose your job?
   c) behind with your work/revision?
   d) unhappy or under too much/little pressure at work?

3. Props – do you:
a) rely on cigarettes/drink/other to get you through the day?
b) get comments about the large amount of alcohol you drink?
c) eat a junky diet, or not have much interest in food?
d) drink as many as 6 or more coffees or colas a day?

4. Health – do you:
a) get a lot of headaches?
b) suffer from nervous stomach upsets?
c) hardly ever get a regular 6–8 hours sleep a night?
d) avoid exercise and other physical activity?

5. Emotions – are you:
a) prone to going 'berserk' when things go wrong for you?
b) easily irritated, even by small things?
c) anxious or worrying about something most of the time?
d) feeling under pressure from boy/girlfriend, home, school or elsewhere?

Your score
Score 0 for each No; for each Yes score the following:
1. a) 2, b) 1, c) 2, d) 2
2. a) 3, b) 6, c) 3, d) 4
3. a) 5, b) 6, c) 3, d) 4
4. a) 4, b) 4, c) 3, d) 4
5. a) 5, b) 2, c) 4, d) 3

Total score = _____

What your score means
Your score is an indication of how well you are coping with stress, that is to say whether you are over-reacting. There are two ways of dealing with stress: internally and externally. Making 'internal' improvements means changing your attitudes and habitual

responses; external ways involve changes to your environment, such as going to bed earlier or improving your diet.

Score 0–10 Some people might say you have an old (mature) head on young shoulders. You are coping well during these turbulent teenage years. Make sure you maintain your positive outlook and stay physically fit and healthy by eating a good diet and exercising. You are in a good position to work hard and achieve a lot while also enjoying yourself to the full.

Score 11–20 With a little bit of effort you could become happier and more relaxed. Take a look at avoidable stresses in your life and try to eliminate them. Try to better understand your emotions and those of family and friends. Take steps to improve your diet and take enough exercise. Find a relaxation technique (meditation, yoga, stretch and tone classes, swimming) that you can practise regularly, and you will soon find that you feel more relaxed and confident about yourself, your appearance and your future.

Score 21–40 You need to take practical steps now to alter your personal habits so that you eat better, sleep better and exercise more. Working all of these changes into your routine will greatly improve your vitality and stamina, and reduce anxiety. If you feel reluctant to change, consider that it is a lot easier to change your habits than change the world (even if the world could do with radical modifications). In other words, life is, to a certain extent, about compromise. So take stock, write down realistic medium-term goals, and learn to express your feelings and needs openly and without hostility.

Score 41+ Reducing stress in your life – and your reactions to situations that are stressful for you – is going to involve quite a bit of work gaining greater insight into your own character and personality. Learning to accept responsibility for your problems and behaviour is important, as well as modifying your quick, often heated, responses. This will mean a combination of reorganizing your lifestyle and making a big effort to change and reduce your reliance on social props. You really are going to have to take a deep breath and count to ten to stop you flying off the handle, before you get into serious trouble. At the top end of the scale (55+) you are probably going to need counselling and other advice to sort out long-held feelings of resentment and difficulty in personal relationships. (See Where to find help page 177.)

Lowering your stress levels

Increased stress from whatever source (family problems, school, exams, work and social pressures) increases your body's demands for vitamins and minerals. In particular, stress increases the demands for B vitamins and the antioxidant vitamins beta-carotene, C and E. Stress can also depress the immune system which a balanced diet can counteract.

You also need to find ways of avoiding stressful situations and ways of coping with stress when it arises. Obviously you can't avoid going to school or work, and in most cases you will not want to leave home! But if you need outside help, see Where to find help, for specialist organisations and agencies.

Teenage stress beaters

- **Take a bath**
  Put some lavender oil (or your favourite bath product) in it for a relaxing soak. Don't have the water too hot and don't wallow too long. Then wrap up warm and relax, or go to bed.
- **Have a good cry or laugh**
  Both are excellent ways of releasing pent-up emotions. Read a tear-jerker book or sob into your pillow; see a soppy movie; watch your favourite comedy video; or get your friends round for a giggle or shoulder to cry on.
- **Talk to someone if possible,**
  talk through your problems in a calm way with your parent(s) or your best friend, or perhaps with a teacher if that seems

appropriate. A teacher might act as an 'arbitrator' if a person at school is giving you grief, or might arrange for you to move down/up a class/set if you are stressed because school work is too difficult/easy.

- **Go for a walk/cycle ride/swim**
  Time on your own while taking a brisk walk or some other exercise will work wonders. An exercise session should leave you feeling exhausted but happy!

- **Have an early night**
  Getting enough rest is important when you are growing and when you have a lot of emotional issues to deal with.

- **Dance away stress**
  If you can, go to a party or a club or anywhere else where you can have a really lively dance session with some friends.

- **Try deep breathing**
  The old advice to count to ten and take deep breaths still holds good when faced with stressful situations. Deep breathing controls stress caused by hyperventilation (short shallow breathing that we do under stress).

- **Listen to music**
  Your mind often sorts things out when you are half-concentrating on music or in a meditative state that can be induced by music.

Reducing stress in the home

Providing a structured environment at home will remove many of the stresses felt by teenagers in coping with homework and exams.

Many parents, and mums in particular, might (half-jokingly) complain that they feel as though they are running a hotel for non-paying guests (eg teenagers) who in some instances are not very appreciative of the five-star service they are receiving. Yet providing regular meals and a space for teenagers to do homework or study undisturbed is vital. Taking the worry out of where the next meal is coming from, and planning a menu that incorporates lots of healthy foods that will aid vitality and brain power – as well as some favourite treats – will allow young minds to concentrate on the learning process.

Providing help and emotional support is also essential. Assisting with planning a revision and study timetable before exams will be very useful (if the school/college does not impart these study skills), but doing the work is out of the question because it is the teenager who has to pass the exams or who should really be doing the continuous assessment units. However, if they are in real difficulty with their schoolwork there is a time when parents should step in and help their teenager express concerns to the school or college.

Most important, let teenagers know that while you expect them to do their best, their results will not affect your love or support for them in whatever they do next.

Incidentally, parents do not have to be chambermaids in their own hotels. Part of the bargain with teenagers is that they keep their rooms clean, make their beds and so on. Although this in itself can become a highly contentious issue, it is not dangerous or anti-social enough to come to blows about!

Cheers! A guide to healthy drinking

Starting to drink alcohol is seen as a 'normal' part of growing up. It is legal to buy beer, cider or perry with a meal in licensed premises from age 16 and legal to buy alcohol from a bar or off licence from age 18. Because alcohol is so widely accepted it is easy to forget that alcohol is actually a drug. Few adults would recognise that fact, so it is hardly surprising that teenagers do not consider drinking risky, like for example taking drugs. Yet doctors (who see the consequences of drinking) think it is.

Our false sense of security with alcohol stems, in part, from the drinks industry, which (with the tacit support of the government) promotes 'sensible drinking' and is very keen to label anyone who takes a radically different view of alcohol as a 'killjoy'. Alcohol, like the National Lottery, is officially labelled 'fun'.

All this is not to say that teenagers (and adults) who are legally old enough should not drink (or buy lottery tickets), but instead to point out that teenagers need to be aware of some of the facts about alcohol that are not yet common currency. Indeed, parents should know these too. As a spokesman for Alcohol Concern has said: 'Before we can educate our children [about drink], we have to educate their parents.'

Things teenagers (and parents) should know about drinking

- Drinking and driving is lethal, and illegal over 80 milligrams of alcohol per 100 millilitres of blood or 35 micrograms of breath. Driving ability is affected by even one drink.
- In America alcoholic drinks have to carry a health warning the same as cigarettes.
- While relaxing inhibitions, alcohol does not improve sexual performance. It impairs performance (ever heard of brewers' droop?).
- More importantly, alcohol can make it very hard for teenagers (girls in particular) to say 'No' to sex, when without the influence of alcohol they would most definitely say 'No'. If the alcohol is flowing you might end up doing something you will bitterly regret.
- Drinking is also related to taking drugs. Many are tried for the first time after alcohol has reduced natural caution. Alcohol is described as the 'gateway' to drug taking.
- Far from making men 'macho', alcohol has a detrimental effect on fertility, reducing men's sperm count (see box) – which, before you ask, does not make it an effective contraceptive!
- Even a very small amount of alcohol can alter your mood. It

Male fertility

If men's semen continues to decline at the present rate, men will be infertile within 60 years, say researchers. Studies on British, French and Danish men show that semen quality is falling. In the British study, men born in 1970 had sperm counts a quarter lower than those born in 1959. Causes are not known for certain, but the strongest theory is that the foetus in the womb is affected by chemicals given off by modern plastics (eg certain food wraps) and pesticide residues in food. Long periods of driving and sitting, also inhibit sperm production by excess warmth.

intensifies emotions which may result in your feeling happy and relaxed, but it can also make you feel depressed.

- Alcohol is high in calories without being high in vitamins and minerals. It also makes extra demands on the body's supplies of vitamin C, B vitamins, zinc and magnesium which are needed to detoxify it, because to the body it is a poisonous drug.
- Alcohol is dehydrating which makes skin lose its elasticity and youthful lustre. Studies have shown that women who drink more than 10 glasses of wine a week, or the equivalent, are more likely to get wrinkles and get them earlier.
- Alcohol makes you urinate more than normal leading to zinc and vitamin losses.
- Alcohol decreases fertility in women.
- Alcohol makes you stupid (like other drugs, it deludes you into thinking you are being smart). It also kills brain cells which cannot be replaced.
- Alcohol kills liver cells, making women in particular more likely to get cirrhosis.
- Adolescents go into a life-threatening coma at lower levels of blood alcohol than adults. (Hence a call by some doctors to

reduce the allowable blood-alcohol levels for teenage drivers. A high proportion of traffic deaths among teenagers are related to alcohol.)

Too much too soon

In Britain one in 25 11- to 15-year-old boys and girls drink more than the maximum amount recommended for adults (see below). More than one in five 13-year-old boys and more than one in eight 13-year-old girls have been 'very drunk' once or more in the previous year. Violent behaviour among teenagers when drunk is common. One in three 15-year-old boys and one in five 15-year-old girls have got into fights and arguments after drinking.

Recommended 'safe' limits for drinking:

Women no more than 14 units a week
Men no more than 21 units a week
(This has recently been revised by the government to 21 units for women and 28 for men – against medical advice and probably under pressure from the drinks industry.)

What is a unit?

One unit = 284ml (½pt) ordinary strength beer, lager or cider 3.5% ABV (Alcohol by Volume, the strength of the drink which appears on the label)
One unit = 1 small glass (125ml) wine 8% ABV
One unit = 1 single pub measure in England and Wales (25ml) spirits 40% ABV. In Northern Ireland a pub measure = 1½ units; in Scotland = 11/4–1½ units.
One unit = 1 small glass (50ml) sherry or port 20% ABV

Teenagers are being unfairly targeted by drinks companies to try to get them hooked sooner, just as tobacco companies now concentrate on selling cigarettes to teenagers and Third World countries, both seen as the most vulnerable markets (older people have wised-up to the weed, and most wish they had never started). There are subtle ways of doing this and subtle advertisements! Some are so subtle that we do not even think about them. For example, on soaps and other television programmes drinking is seen as being pleasurable, even socially desirable. No-one wants to be the odd one out.

Then there are the subtle advertisements that use teenagers and young people slightly older than the market they are aiming for, to depict to younger teenagers the image that drinking is expected and accepted behaviour for normal young adults. And in addition, that drinking is fun and sociable and wins the approval of peers. Clever stuff.

So clever that doctors and others are constantly calling on government to put in place tighter controls on advertising and marketing aimed at the young (including sponsorship of the arts and sports events by alcohol companies). And consumer groups want the number of alcohol units to be put on labels of alcoholic drinks so that everyone can see how much they are drinking. For example, a bottle of regular beer/lager might contain 1–1½ units of alcohol compared with 2 or more in a bottle of 'special' beer.

Some observers might think that government puts drinks companies and its purse before the concerns for health and welfare of teenagers (who are not, after all, contributing any taxes, and may not yet be able to vote). This view is reinforced by the government allowing drinks companies to sell mineral water, cola, lemonade, cherryades and other 'children's drinks' laced with alcohol. The taste of alcohol is masked completely, so that the soft drinks are acceptable to teenagers – and younger children.

If you are going to drink, here's how to do it

Drinking is undeniably pleasurable for most people, and the key to 'safe and enjoyable' drinking seems to be to drink with food – when you are not going to drive afterwards. Regard alcohol (ie wine and beer) as part of a meal. In the Mediterranean countries – France, Italy, Greece, Spain and Portugal – the traditional pattern of drinking is moderate amounts with food. There they have far fewer social problems with alcohol, and there are some health benefits as far as heart disease is concerned.

In Britain (and Germany, the Netherlands, Scandinavia, Canada and Australia), beer drinking seems to promote a 'bravado' culture, where getting drunk and getting into fights are a normal part of adolescent (and older) recreation. Beer is, of course, drunk without food, which would modify its effects.

Smoking – giving up without putting on weight

Although more teenagers are smoking, it is no longer seen as rebellious and trendy. And even though more teenagers are smoking, they are also nagging their parents to give up. So why do they smoke?

Teenagers – and young children – start to smoke for all sorts of reasons
- there are smokers at home
- pressure from friends to join in
- curiosity which leads to getting hooked
- it's not allowed.

Whatever the reason, we all now know that it is not a good idea to smoke because of the risks of heart disease and cancer from smoking. Of course the risk of disease later in life is rarely a deterrent during the teen years. Then there is a wonderful feeling of immortality and optimism about being the exception to the rule, who can smoke (and/or drink and lounge around) and still live to be a ripe old age. Teenagers may also take the popular (if erroneous) view that risky hobbies are a part of normal life, and that you are just as likely to be run over by a bus tomorrow, so hang the consequences of today's actions.

But even if long-term health is not a concern, smoking has some very unpleasant effects:

- Smoking makes you smelly. Your clothes, hair and hands will stink of cigarettes.
- Smoking makes you less attractive. Fingers and teeth, and eventually the whites of the eyes, will be stained yellow.
- Smoking makes you sound repulsive. Probably no-one in the known universe has ever found a smoker's cough a turn-on.
- Smoking makes you ill more often. You will get more coughs, colds and other infections because your lungs can't work properly as they are filled with effluent (tar) and phlegm. Smoking doubles your needs for vitamin C (which protects against colds and far worse infections) and B vitamins.
- Smokers get earlier on-set of wrinkles.
- Smokers will soon be addicted. Doctors say smoking is a harder addiction to kick than heroin. Even if smokers think they can stop whenever they want to, they can't. Ask adult smokers who have given up – innumerable times.
- Smokers have less money to spend on clothes, hairdressers, cds, going out, books …
- Smokers who smoke to keep slim have to ask themselves if there isn't an easier way to do it. (There is, as this book shows.) They can be slim – and healthy and more attractive for all of the above reasons.

Making yourself a smoke-free zone

Smoking is on the decline in the UK, except among 16- to 24-year-old women, more of whom are smoking than ever before. It is estimated that 17% of 16-year-old females and 19% of males are regular smokers, rising to 24% and 22% 17-year-olds respectively. If you are fed up with parents, friends and teachers, all nagging you to give up, or sick of being a social outcast at work – forced to have a fag outside the building – then you probably need new motivation help to give up, especially if surveys are true that say 90% of 16-to 19-year-old smokers would like to give up, but don't have the motivation.

Special diet needs of smokers

Studies comparing the diets of teenage smokers with those of never or occasional smokers show that teenage girls, in particular, have a very different diet from non-smokers. They have a significantly lower intake of antioxidant nutrients (vitamin C, carotene, folic acid, zinc, selenium), fruits, vegetables and cereals.

Both male and female teenage smokers are less likely to eat wholemeal bread and sweet foods such as puddings and biscuits. Both male and female smokers drink significantly more alcohol than non-smokers, and more coffee, and eat more chips and processed meats. The result is that smokers have a diet higher in fat and lower in fibre. Smokers in general also eat foods with fewer B vitamins and iron, and teenage girl smokers consume less protein and calcium.

Help with giving up

Advice from counsellors on how to quit, and support while you do so, are available from Quit. The organisation also has a pack of eight postcards with humorous, startling and gory images on the front, and hard-hitting facts on the consequences of smoking on the back. The Break Free postcard pack was designed by young people for young people, who said 'don't patronise us, don't lie to us, don't preach to us, just give us the facts in straightforward language with strong visual images'. See if it works for you. It's available free from the Quitline on 0800 00 22 00, free of charge, between 9.30am and 5.30pm any day of the week.

Quit without weight gain

Not everyone puts on weight when they stop smoking. For those who do, it is usually only a few pounds which can be lost within a matter of months, once you are feeling more comfortable with the way you look and eat. The reason some people put on a bit of weight is that smoking depresses the appetite and reduces the sensation of taste. The body also burns calories trying to detoxify itself from the poisonous by-products of smoking. The main thing is to be positive. You will be healthier and look better once you have given up, and you will be able to control your weight through exercise and diet. You probably will not have to eat less – just differently.

Stop smoking, mum

Even teenagers who smoke try to get their parents to give up.

Allergic to food?

Most 'bad reactions' to food are caused by food poisoning, but around 2% of the population may be allergic to a food, or have a food intolerance or sensitivity.

A food allergy involves the immune system reacting inappropriately to food, or an additive or ingredient in food. Food intolerance, sometimes called 'false food allergies', can provoke the same symptoms as an allergy, but without involving the immune system.

Often food intolerance is due to the body lacking a particular enzyme needed to digest a food. For example, people who cannot digest lactose (the naturally occurring sugars in milk), lack the enzyme lactase. This is not an allergic reaction.

An adverse reaction to food can occur in minutes, or develop over several hours. Typical symptoms include: swollen lips, tingling mouth, vomiting, abdominal distension and pain, diarrhoea.

If it is known that you are in danger of severe allergic reaction,

---

WARNING

Anyone who suffers a severe allergic reaction is in danger of going into anaphylactic shock, which causes difficulty breathing and swelling inside and around the mouth and throat, carrying a risk of suffocation. Call an ambulance immediately. Until help arrives, support the person in the position that most helps their breathing. Loosen clothing at the neck and waist. If the person loses consciousness, put them in the recovery position and be prepared to resuscitate. Check if they have adrenaline medication on them.

---

your doctor may provide you with a syringe of adrenaline for use in emergencies, should you accidentally eat the substance to which you are allergic.

The foods that most commonly cause allergic reactions are: eggs, dairy produce, wheat-based cereal, strawberries, fish and shellfish. Sensitivity to cow's milk protein is fairly common in young children – up to 10% may experience it. Usually it disappears by the time children are at primary school.

Are you allergic?

If you suspect a food allergy (or intolerance), consult your GP. Food allergy is more common in people who suffer other forms of allergy or hypersensitivity, eg asthma, allergic rhinitis (hay fever) and eczema. Food allergies can also contribute to these conditions.

It is important to seek help from your GP or dietitian (either GP or hospital-based) before excluding foods from your diet. If you try to self-diagnose a food allergy, there is a danger – especially with children – that too many restrictions might be imposed, leaving the body short of essential nutrients. Your GP might suggest a process of elimination, such as a food diary, to work out foods to which you might be allergic. Some GPs arrange more scientific diagnostic tests for food allergy.

The usual diagnostic test involves patches soaked with substances suspected of causing the allergy being taped to the skin (often on the back). Alternatively, the substances may be injected just below the surface of the skin. When the patches are removed, or where the skin has been pricked, the allergy-producing substances leave inflamed red area. The tests are not infallible, and red areas may occur with substances to which you are not allergic.

Treating food allergy

The only treatment for food allergy is to avoid the offending food. Desensitization, which involves giving minute, but increasing, doses of the substance at fault to promote tolerance, used to be a popular treatment. But low success rates have resulted in this treatment being abandoned.

It is important to learn to live with your food allergy because it may be lifelong and irreversible – even life threatening.

What to do

- Learn all the synonyms (other names) for the food or food ingredient so that you can see it when reading food labels.
- Question staff in food shops where food is unlabelled, and do not buy if they do not know the exact ingredients.
- Ask in restaurants and cafés if a particular dish on the menu contains the food to which you are allergic. It may only be a garnish and therefore not listed in the description of the dish given on the menu.

What causes an allergic reaction?

A true food allergy will cause the body to produce antibodies. Antibodies are proteins that neutralise antigens. Antigens are foreign proteins (viruses and bacteria) that trigger production of antibodies. In a food allergy the food, or a substance in it, acts as an antigen to trigger a particular type of antibody attached to mast cells. Once activated the mast cells release powerful substances such as histamine

---

Not in bread alone...

Many foods are found in unexpected places. Wheat (and other grains), for example, are not only found in bread and breakfast cereals. They are also used as thickeners, in breaded foods, as fillers in stock cubes, in snack foods, in stuffing, in batters, and in pastry and pies. In disguise, wheat occurs as modified starch in dairy food such as yogurt and desserts, and as rusk in sausages and other meat products. Beers can also be brewed partly from wheat.

---

and prostaglandins, which cause the inflammation or sudden drop in blood pressure associated with an allergic reaction.

In false food allergies and some forms of food intolerance, people may suffer similar symptoms but not be truly allergic, because the offending foods trigger mast cells to produce histamine, but antibodies are not involved. That is why only laboratory tests can determine whether a food allergy is true or false.

All in the family

Allergic conditions such as hay fever, asthma and eczema tend to run in families. This condition is described as atopy, and people with classic allergic symptoms are described as atopic. As atopy is often inherited, it may be that the genes responsible for immune control are acting abnormally.

Common food allergies

Food allergies tend to be confined to very specific food groups.

Nut allergies You can be allergic to peanuts, but not to other nuts. The peanut is a member of the legume family (beans, peas and lentils). It is the lectins in legumes that cause an allergic reaction. (These are also the substances that need to be boiled to inactivate them when cooking kidney and haricot beans. Inactivated they can cause serious diarrhoea.)

Wheat allergies may be either to gluten in wheat (also found in other grains such as rye, barley and oats) or to lectins or other components found in wheat.

Shellfish (prawns, shrimps, crabs, lobsters) Protein-like substances in shellfish, called peptides (also found in eggs, strawberries, tomatoes, fish, pork and chocolate), are thought to be responsible for the bad reactions they cause.

Special diet food products

Egg replacers, wheat-free pasta and bread, gluten-free bread mixes and lactose-free dairy foods can be obtained from pharmacies and health food shops and from specialist suppliers, some of which offer mail order. Supermarkets produce lists of products that can be eaten by people with certain allergies, plus information leaflets; contact customer relations departments.

CHAPTER 9

Where to find help

How to seek help or information for personal problems.

Going to the doctor

Even if you are under 16, doctors still have to keep anything you tell them private, just as they would for an adult. This might come as a surprise when you are not used to having what you say to someone being treated 'in confidence'. So whether you ask for advice about a cold, or contraception or a sexual problem, or worries about drink or drugs, or eating disorders or depression, your doctor will not tell anyone else (including parents and teachers) what has been discussed (unless the doctor is concerned enough about your 'competency' to deal with the situation to reveal information 'in your best interest'). You do not need your parent's permission to see a doctor, and you can make an appointment to see a doctor without your parent(s) accompanying you. However, it is best if you can talk to your parents about all issues, including those that you might want to see the doctor about, for example if you are thinking of starting, or have already started, having sex. Your doctor may suggest you talk to your parents.

If you have doubts, ring the doctor's surgery and ask if confidential advice will be given to under-16-year-olds. If it is not, or if you want contraceptive services and your doctor's practice does not offer these, then you could either ask your GP to refer you to another doctor or doctor's clinic where contraceptive services are available (without having to change your main doctor), or you can go to a local family planning clinic (see telephone numbers below). You can also change doctors from the age of 16, if you want to.

Action Against Allergy
24-26 High Street
Hampton Hill, Middx TW12 1PD
Send large sae for list of information leaflets available and general guidance. Newsletter also available.

AIDS/HIV and sexually transmitted diseases
National AIDS Helpline
0800 567123 (24 hours)
Terrence Higgins Trust
0171 242 1010 (12noon-10pm daily)

British Allergy Foundation
St Bartholemew's Hospital
London EC1A 7BE
Send large sae for further information. Helpline planned.

British Complementary Medicine Association
39 Prestbury Road
Cheltenham, Glos GL52 2PT
01242 226 770 (Mon–Fri 10am–4pm)
Register of complementary practitioners and contacts; small donations (from 50p) requested.

British Heart Foundation
14 Fitzhardinge Street
London W1H 4DH
0171 935 0185
Send sae for information on prevention of heart disease – which affects women as well as men – and other aspects of heart health.

British Pregnancy Advice Service
Head Office: Austy Manor
Wootton Wawen
Solihull, West Midlands B95 6BX
BPAS Actionline 0345 304 030
BPAS provides confidential friendly advice, treatment and support in the areas of unplanned pregnancy and fertility control. For further information and appointment at any of BPAS' 30 consultation centres nationwide call the Actionline (above)

Brook Advisory Centre
165 Gray's Inn Road
London WC1X 8UD
0171 713 9000 (Mon-Fri 9am–4.30pm)
0171 617 8000 (24-hour recorded information Helpline)
Offers teenagers free confidential contraceptive advice and supplies, and help with emotional and sexual problems. There are free pregnancy tests and staff available to discuss continuing the pregnancy or referral for abortion. For details of regional centres contact the above telephone/address.

Careline
0181 514 1177
Britain's only telephone counselling service
that offers 24-hour advice, information and
counselling on any issue

Child Growth Foundation
2 Mayfield Avenue
London W4 1PW
0181 995 0257
Charity concerned with child growth
and publishers of UK current national
growth standards.

ChildLine 0800 1111
ChildLine is the free confidential
national helpline for children in trouble
or danger. It provides a telephone
counselling service for any child with
any problem, 24 hours a day, every day.

Children's Legal Centre
0120 687 3820 (Mon–Fri 2pm–5pm)
Offers free legal advice for young people.

Defeat Depression Campaign
The Royal College of Psychiatrists
17 Belgrave Square
London SW1X 8PG
0171 235 2351
A national campaign organised by family
doctors and psychiatrists.

Eating Disorders Association
Sackville Place
44-48 Magdalen Street
Norwich
Norfolk NR3 IJU
Helpline 01603 621414
(Mon-Fri 9am-6.30pm)
Youth Helpline (18 years and under)
01603 765050
(Mon-Fri 9am-6.30pm)
Recorded message about anorexia
nervosa and bulimia nervosa
0891 615466
The Eating Disorders Association offers
help and support to people with
anorexia nervosa and bulimia nervosa
and their families and friends.

Eating for Pregnancy Helpline
Wellbeing Centre for Pregnancy and
Nutrition
University of Sheffield
Northern General Hospital
Herries Road
Sheffield S5 7AU
0114 242 4084
Telephone advice for healthy eating
before, during and after pregnancy.
Leaflets available.

Family Planning Association

For information on contraception, sexual and reproductive health care, details of your nearest family planning clinic and free leaflets, from:

(England)
27-35 Mortimer Street
London W1N 7RJ
(Mon-Fri 9am-5pm)
0171 6363 7866

(Northern Ireland)
113 University Street
Belfast BT7 1HP
(Mon-Fri 9am-5pm)
01232 325488

(Wales)
4 Museum Place
Cardiff CF1 3BG
(Mon-Fri 9am-5pm)
01222 342766

(Scotland)
2 Claremont Terrace
Glasgow G3 7XR
(Mon-Fri 9am-5pm)
0141 211 8138

Folic Acid (and planning a pregnancy) information

Health Information Service free phone:
0800 665 544

Foresight

The Association for the Promotion of Preconceptual Care
28 The Paddock
Godalming, Surrey GU7 1XD
Send sae for dietary and other preconceptual information.

Lakeland Plastics Ltd

Alexandra Buildings, Windermere
Cumbria LA23 1BQ
01539 488300
Mail order catalogue of equipment for home-made iced lollies, milk shakes, and other cookery and food preparation and storage equipment.

Maternity Alliance Helpline

0171 588 8582 (Mon–Fri 10am–1pm)

Mindline 0800 110 100

Radio One's 24-hour free telephone line for free confidential help and advice.

National Association for Premenstrual Syndrome (NAPS)

PO Box 72
Sevenoaks,
Kent TN13 1XQ
01732 741709

National Children's Bureau

8 Wakely Street
London EC1V 7QE
0171 843 6000

National Drugs Helpline 0800 776 600

Free and confidential service which gives advice and information to callers with concerns or questions about drugs. The line also provides counselling to callers with drug-related problems.

National Osteoporosis Society

PO Box 10
Radstock,
Bath BA3 3YB
01761 471771
Send sae for information.

NCH Action for Children
85 Highbury Park
London N5 1UD
0171 226 2033
Regional centres for mums and babies
and has a selection of literature.
Information on additional benefits and
free milk from Citizens Advice Bureaux,
local council offices or local Benefits
Agency office (all in the Yellow Pages).
For help on maternity rights contact:

Quit Helpline 0800 002 200
(9.30am-5.30pm)
Victory House
170 Tottenham Court Road
London W1P 0HA
Support and helpline for those wishing
to give up smoking.

Release
388 Old Street
London EC1V 9LT
0171 729 9904
Advice and referral on drug and legal
problems, and emergency help in the
case of arrest.

The Samaritans
0345 909 090
Provides emotional support to depressed
and suicidal people, 24 hours a day.

The School Meals Campaign
PO Box 402
London WC1H 9TZ
0171 383 7638

Sports Nutrition Foundation
National Sports Medical Institute
c/o Medical College,
St Bartholemews
Charterhouse Square
London EC1M 6BQ

Trust for the Study of Adolescence
23 New Road
Brighton,
East Sussex BN1 1WZ
01273 693 311
Tapes and books for teenagers, parents
and those who work with adolescents.

The Vegetarian Society
Parkdale
Dunham Road
Altrincham, Cheshire WA14 4QG
0161 928 0793
Offers advice for vegetarians on food
and nutrition. Please send sae.

The Vegan Society
7 Battle Road
St Leonards-on-Sea,
East Sussex TN37 7AA
01424 427393

APPENDIX

Additives

Colourings: E120 (cochineal colouring), E153 (carbon black, although there is a vegetable carbon), E161g (canthaxanthin, a colouring from shells.

Preservatives: E203 calcium sorbate, E213 calcium benzoate, E227 calcium hydrogen sulphate (and others), 234 nisin, E263 calcium acetate, E270 lactic acid, E282 calcium propionate, 297 fumaric acid.

Antioxidants: E302 calcium L-ascorbate, E304 6-0-palmitoyl-L-ascorbic acid.

Emulsifiers, stabilisers, thickeners: E322 lecithin, E325 sodium lactate, E326 potassium lactate, E327 calcium lactate, E333 monoCalcium citrate (and others), E334 tartaric acid, E338 orthophosporic acid, E339 sodium dihydrogen orthophosphate (and others), E 340 potassium dihydrogen orthophosphate (and others), E341 calcium tetrahydrogen diorthophosphate (and others), 352 calcium malate, E404 calcium alginate.

Synthetic sweeteners: E422 glycerol, 430 polyoxyethylene (8) stearate, 431 polyoxyethylene (40) stearate, 432 polyoxyethylene (20) sorbitan monolaurate (polysorbate 20), 433 polyoxyethylene (20) sorbitan mono-oleate (polysorbate 80), 434 polyoxyethylene (20) sorbitan monopalmitate (polysorbate 40), 435 polyoxyethylene (20) sorbitan monostearate (polysorbate 60), 436 polyoxyethylene (20) sorbitan tristearate (polysorbate 65).

Emulsifiers stabilisers, thickeners: E450 (a) tetraPotassium diphosphate, E450(b) tetraPotassium triphosphate, E450(c) sodium polyphosphates (and others), E470 sodium, potassium and calcium salts of fatty acids, E471 mono- and di-glyercides of fatty acids, E472(a) acetic acid esters of mono- and di-glycerides of fatty acids, E472(b) lactic acid esters of mono-and di-glycerides of fatty acids (Lactoglycerides), E472 (c) citric acid esters of mono- and di-glycerides of fatty acids (citroglycerides), E472(e) mono- and diacetyltartaric acid esters of mono- and di-glycerides of fatty acids, E473 sucrose esters of fatty acids, E474 sucroglycerides, E475 polyglycerol esters of fatty acids, E477 propane-1,2-diol esters of fatty acids, 478 lactylated fatty acid esters of glycerol and propane-1,2-diol, E481 sodium stearolyl-2-lacylate, E482 calcium stearolyl-2-lacylate, E483 stearyl tartrate, 491 sorbitan monostearate, 492 sorbitan tristearate.

Anti-caking agents: 542 edible bone phosphate, 570 stearic acid, 572 magnesium stearate.

Flavour enhancers, sweeteners: 627 guanosine 5'-(disodium phosphate) (sodium guanylate), 631 Inosine 5'-(disodium phosphate) (sodium inosinate).

Glazing agents: 901 beeswax, 904 shellac.

Improving, bleaching agents: 92- L-cysteine hydrochloride.

Sweeteners: aspartame.

Miscellaneous: glycine, oxystearine.

Selected bibliography

1. *The National Food Guide, The Balance of Good Health* (1994) Health Education Authority in partnership with the Department of Health and the Ministry of Agriculture, Fisheries and Food

2. *Diet, nutrition and the prevention of chronic diseases* (1990) report of a World Health Organization Study Group

3. *Nutritional Aspects of Coronary Heart Disease* (1994) report of Committee on Medical Aspects of Food Policy

4. *Dietary Reference Values for Food energy and Nutrients for the UK* (1991) report of the panel on Dietary Reference Values of the Committee on Medical Aspects of Food Policy

5. *Enjoy Healthy Eating*, Health Education Authority, 1995

6. 'Dietary habits of 15- to 25-year-olds', Nicola L Bull, *Human Nutrition: Applied Nutrition* (1985), 39a supplement 1:1-68

7. 'The nutrient and food intakes of 16- to 17-year-old female dieters in the UK' by Helen Crawley and Rita Shergill-Bonner, *Journal of Human Nutrition and Dietetics* (1995), 8, 25-34

8. *The Diets of British Schoolchildren* (1986) preliminary report of a nutritional analysis of a nationwide dietary survey of British schoolchildren by RW Wenlock, MM Disselduff and RK Skinner, Department of Health and Social Security, and I Knight, Office of Population Censuses and Surveys

9. 'The role of breakfast cereals in the diets of 16- to 17-year-old teenagers in Britain', Helen Crawley, *Journal of Human Nutrition and Dietetics* (1993), 6, 205-216

10. 'The energy, nutrient and food intakes of teenagers aged 16-17 years in Britain', Helen Crawley, *British Journal of Nutrition* (1993), 70, 15-26

11. 'The diet and body weight of British teenage smokers at 16-17 years', HF Crawley and D While, *European Journal of Clinical Nutrition* (1995), 49, 904-914

12. 'Standard from birth to maturity for height, weight, height velocity and weight velocity: British Children', *Archives of Disease in Childhood* (1966), 41:454-471

13. 'Body mass index reference curves for the UK', 1990, T J Cole, J V Freeman, MA Preece, *Archives of Disease in Childhood* (1995), 73:25-29

14. 'Foods eaten outside the home: nutrient contribution to total diet', J M Loughridge, A D Walker, H Sarsby and R Shepherd, *Journal of Human Nutrition and Dietetics* (1989), 2:361-369

15. *Physical Activity Strategy Statement, Physical Activity Task Force,* (1996), Department of Health

16. 'Long term health implications of fitness and physical activity patterns', C Riddoch, J M Savage, N Murphy, G W Cran, C Boreham, *Archives of Disease in Childhood* (1991), 66: 1426-1433

17. *Children's Exercise, Health and Fitness* (1988), Sports Council

18. *Medical Aspects of Exercise: benefits and risks* (1991), report of the Royal College of Physicians

19. *Allied Dunbar National Fitness Survey* (1993) in conjunction with the Health Education Authority, Sports Council and Look After Your Heart

20. *The Royal College of General Practitioners, conference on adolescent care in practice,* 1995

21. 'Teen-zine sex is not all it seems', *British Medical Journal* (1996), 312:451

22. 'Teenage sex, cognitive immaturity increases the risks', *British Medical Journal* (1996), 312:390-391

23. 'Alcohol and the Young' (1995) a report by the British Paediatric Association and the Royal College of Physicians

24. *Health Promotion and the family: messages from four research studies,* (1996), Health Education Authority

25. *The Use of Very Low Calorie Diets in Obesity* (1987) report of the Working Group on Very Low Calorie Diets, Committee on Medical Aspects of Food Policy, Department of Health and Social Security

26. *Obesity* (1983) a report of the Royal College of Physicians

27. *Obesity: reversing the Increasing Problem of Obesity in England* (1995) a report from the Nutrition and Physical Activity Task Forces, The Health of the Nation

28. *Exploding the Myths of Obesity* (1995) symposium organised by the Association for the Study of Obesity, St Bartholomew's Hospital, London

29. *The Health of the Nation, a strategy for health in England,* 1992

30. *Health Survey for England 1993,* Office of Population Census and Surveys

31. *On the State of the Public Health, 1994,* the annual report of the Chief Medical Officer of Health, Department of Health

32. *Living in Britain, 1994 General Household Survey,* Office of Population Censuses and Surveys

33. *The Health of the Young Nation conference, London 1995,* organised by the Department of Health with participation from the Departments for Education and Transport

34. *The Nation's Diet Conference* (1995), Economic & Social Research Council research programme, London

35. *Nutritional Guidelines for School Meals,* (1992) report of an Expert Working Group, The Caroline Walker Trust,

36. *The Nutritional Case for School Meals* (1992) School Meals Campaign

37. *School Meals, take action!* (1992) School Meals Campaign

38. *Healthy School Food: a guide for school governors and school boards* (1994) School Meals Campaign

39. *School Meals Assessment Pack* (1995) National Heart Forum

40. *Diet and Health in School Age Children* (1995) nutrition briefing paper, Health Education Authority

41. *Food for Children, influencing choice and investing in health* (1993) report of conference on Diet and School children organised by the National Forum for Coronary Heart Disease Prevention

42. *Children's Diets and Change (1987) a report of the Child Health and Nutrition Working Party*, The British Dietetic Association

43. *The Gardner Merchant School Meals Survey, 1994*

44. School Dinners, are they worth having?' *Which?* (September 1992), 502-504

45. 'How healthy is your breakfast cereal?' *Which?* (February 1996), 8-13

46. 'Which Way to Health, Are you sure you need to lose weight?' *Which?* (February 1995), 22-24

47. *Young Women and Osteoporosis*, one day meeting of the National Osteoporosis Society, 1995

48. *The Growing Cycle, Child Mother Child (1994)* conference organised by the National Dairy Council, London

49. *Folic Acid and the Prevention of Neural Tube Defects (1992)* report from an expert Advisory Group, Department of Health

50. *Early Diet, Later Consequences*, The British Nutrition Foundation Nutrition Bulletin (1991) 16, supplement 1

51. 'Eating Disorders Review', *The Journal of the Eating Disorders Association,* (1995) 3, 127-196, Dissociation and the Eating Disorders

52. *Eating Disorders '93,* conference and exhibition organised by *British Journal of Hospital Medicine* in association with The Hospital for Sick Children, Great Ormond Street, London, 1993

53. *Vegetarian Vitality* (1995) a report of the health benefits of vegetarian diet and the nutritional requirements of vegetarians, The Vegetarian Society

54. *The Realeat Survey(s) of Meat Eating and Vegetarianism 1987-1995*

55. 'Why we eat what we eat', *The British Nutrition Foundation Nutrition Bulletin* (1990) 15, supplement 1

56. *Eating for Performance (1995) a practical guide*, produced by the Sports Nutrition Foundation

57. *Nutrition and Teenagers*, National Dairy Council (1995) Fact File no 5

58. 'Teenage Eating Habits' *Quarterly Review, National Dairy Council Nutrition Service* (winter 1995) 9-12,

59. *The Threat to our Children's Teeth (1995)* report commissioned by Colgate

60. 'Can children's intelligence be increased by vitamin and mineral supplementation?' *Lancet* (1988) ii, 335

61. *The Liverpool Project (1986)* study of a wholefood nutritional programme in an institutional setting by Liverpool social services department in association with Booker Health

62. *Evolution and Healing, the new science of Darwinian medicine* (1995) Randolph M Nesse & George C Williams (Weidenfeld & Nicolson)

63. *The Driving Force: food, evolution and the future* (1989) Michael Crawford & David Marsh, Heinemann

64. *Healthy Eating on a Plate* (1995) Janette Marshall, Vermilion

65. *The Ultimate ACE Diet: halve your risk of cancer and heart disease* (1994) Janette Marshall, Vermilion

66. *Eat for Life Diet* Janette Marshall and Anne Heughan (1992) Vermilion, (1993) Arrow

Index

Acknowledgements

Dr Bridget Dolan, Chair for the European Council of Eating Disorders, Department of Mental Health Sciences, St George's Medical School, London, for finding time to read and comment on the text, so constructively. Lyndel Costain, BSc SRD State Registered Dietitian, for responses to the teenage eating diaries and comments on the text. Kathy Moyse, whose pupils kindly completed food diaries, plus all the other teenagers who filled in food diaries and gave their thoughts on the book's title and contents – and shared their jokes! Tam Fry, chairman of The Child Growth Foundation. Mr Alan Honson, Assistant Director Coaching and Education (Medical Education), Football Association.